Respiratory Medicine

From our teachers and their teachers,
to our students and their students

LECTURE NOTES ON

Respiratory Medicine

S.J. BOURKE

MD, FRCPI, FCCP, DCH

Consultant Physician
Royal Victoria Infirmary
Newcastle upon Tyne
Senior Lecturer in Medicine
University of Newcastle upon Tyne

R.A.L. BREWIS

MD, FRCP

Emeritus Consultant Physician
Royal Victoria Infirmary
Queen Victoria Road
Newcastle upon Tyne
Senior Lecturer in Medicine
University of Newcastle upon Tyne

Fifth edition

Blackwell
Science

© 1975, 1980, 1985, 1991, 1998 by
Blackwell Science Ltd
Editorial Offices:
Osney Mead, Oxford OX2 0EL
25 John Street, London WC 1N 2BL
23 Ainslie Place, Edinburgh EH3 6AJ
350 Main Street, Malden
    MA 02148 5018, USA
54 University Street, Carlton
    Victoria 3053, Australia
10, rue Casimir Delavigne
    75006 Paris, France

Other Editorial Offices:
Blackwell Wissenschafts-Verlag GmbH
Kurfürstendamm 57
10707 Berlin, Germany

Blackwell Science KK
MG Kodenmacho Building
7–10 Kodenmacho Nihombashi
Chuo-ku, Tokyo 104, Japan

Iowa State University Press
A Blackwell Science Company
2121 S. State Avenue
Ames, Iowa 50014-8300, USA

First published 1975
Second edition 1980
Third edition 1985
Fourth edition 1991
Fifth edition 1998
Reprinted 1999, 2002

Set by Excel Typesetters Co.,
Hong Kong
Printed and bound in Great Britain at
the Alden Press, Oxford and
Northampton

A catalogue record for this title
is available from the British Library

ISBN 0-632-04968-5

Library of Congress
Cataloging-in-publication Data

Bourke, S.J.
    Lecture notes on respiratory
medicine. — 5th ed./S.J. Bourke,
R.A.L. Brewis.
        p.   cm.
    Rev. ed. of: Lecture notes on
respiratory disease/written and
illustrated by R.A.L. Brewis. 4th ed.
1991.
    Includes bibliographical
references and index.
    ISBN 0-632-04968-5
    I. Respiratory organs—Diseases
—Outlines, syllabi, etc. I. Brewis,
R.A.L. II. Title.
    [DNLM: I. Respiratory Tract
Diseases.
WF 140 B774L 1998]
RC731.B69 1998
616.2—dc21
DNLM/DLC
for Library of Congress   98-3473
                                       CIP

DISTRIBUTORS

Marston Book Services Ltd
PO Box 269
Abingdon, Oxon OX14 4YN
(Orders: Tel: 01235 465500
        Fax: 01235 465555)

The Americas
Blackwell Publishing
c/o AIDC
PO Box 20
50 Winter Sport Lane
Williston, VT 05495-0020
(Orders: Tel: 800 216 2522
        Fax: 802 864 7626)

Australia
Blackwell Science Pty Ltd
54 University Street
Carlton, Victoria 3053
(Orders: Tel: 3 9347 0300
        Fax: 3 9347 5001)

For further information on
Blackwell Science, visit our website:
www.blackwell-science.com

The Blackwell Science logo is a
trade mark of Blackwell Science Ltd,
registered at the United Kingdom
Trade Marks Registry

Contents

Preface

The fifth edition of *Lecture Notes on Respiratory Medicine* has been written at a time when respiratory diseases account for a large proportion of acute medical problems presenting to hospitals and general practice, when asthma is increasing in prevalence, when the global threat of tuberculosis is re-emerging and when advances in molecular biology are being translated into clinical practice in diseases such as cystic fibrosis. The text of previous editions has been modified to provide a concise, up-to-date summary of respiratory medicine in line with a modern undergraduate curriculum. It takes into account published guidelines and consensus statements, and will be useful to junior doctors preparing for postgraduate exams and to general physicians undertaking continuing medical education. Above all it remains a patient-based book to be read before and after visits to the wards and clinics where clinical medicine is learnt and practised. We are grateful to our teachers, and their teachers, and we pass on our evolving knowledge of respiratory medicine to our students, and their students.

S.J. Bourke
R.A.L. Brewis

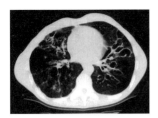

CHAPTER 1

Anatomy and Physiology of the Lungs

Introduction

The essential function of the lungs is the **exchange of oxygen and carbon dioxide between the blood and the atmosphere**. This takes place by a process of molecular diffusion across the alveolar capillary membrane which has a surface area of about 60 m². The anatomy and physiology of the respiratory system are designed in such a way as to bring air from the atmosphere and blood from the circulation into close contact across the alveolar capillary membrane. Contraction of the diaphragm and intercostal muscles results in expansion of the chest and a fall in intrathoracic pressure which draws atmospheric air containing 21% oxygen into the lungs. **Ventilation** of the alveoli depends upon the size of each breath (tidal volume), respiratory rate, resistance of the airways to airflow, and compliance (distensibility) of the lungs. About a quarter of the air breathed in remains in the conducting airways and is not available for gas exchange: this is referred to as the anatomical deadspace. The lungs are **perfused** by almost all the cardiac output from the right ventricle. There is a complex and dynamic interplay between ventilation and perfusion in maintaining gas exchange in health, and derangement of these parameters is a key pathophysiological feature of respiratory disease. Ventilation of alveoli which are not perfused increases deadspace, and blood passing from the pulmonary artery to the left atrium without passing through ventilated alveoli does not contribute to gas exchange, thereby forming a physiological shunt.

Bronchial tree

The **trachea** has cartilaginous horseshoe-shaped 'rings' supporting its anterior and lateral walls. The posterior wall is flaccid and bulges forward during coughing. The trachea divides into the right and left main bronchi at the level of the sternal angle (angle of Louis). The **left main bronchus** is longer than the right and leaves the trachea at a more abrupt angle. The **right main bronchus** is more directly in line with the trachea so that inhaled material tends to enter the right lung more readily than the left. The main bronchi divide into **lobar bronchi** (upper, middle and lower on the right; upper and lower on the left) and then **segmental bronchi** as shown in Fig. 1.1. The position of the lungs in relation to external landmarks is shown in Fig. 1.2. **Bronchi** are airways with cartilage in their walls, and there are about 10 divisions of bronchi beyond the tracheal bifurcation. Smaller airways without cartilage in their walls are referred to as **bronchioles**. **Respiratory bronchioles** are peripheral bronchioles with alveoli in their walls. Bronchioles immediately proximal to alveoli are known as **terminal bronchioles**.

BRONCHOPULMONARY SEGMENTS

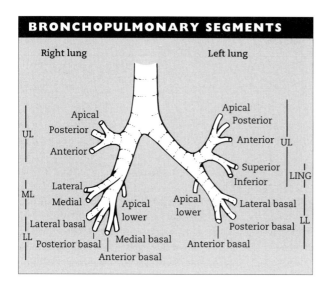

Fig. 1.1 Diagram of bronchopulmonary segments. UL, upper lobe; ML, middle lobe; LL, lower lobe; LING, lingula.

SURFACE ANATOMY OF THE LUNGS

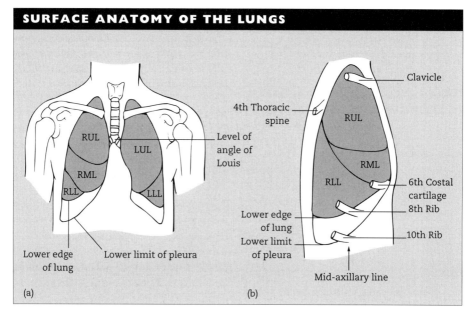

Fig. 1.2 Surface anatomy. (a) Anterior view of the lungs. (b) Lateral view of the right side of chest at resting end-expiratory position. RUL, right upper lobe; RML, right middle lobe; RLL, right lower lobe; LUL, left upper lobe; LLL, left lower lobe.

In the bronchi, smooth muscle is arranged in a spiral fashion internal to the cartilaginous plates. The muscle coat becomes more complete distally as the cartilaginous plates become more fragmentary. The epithelial lining is ciliated and includes goblet cells. The cilia beat with a whip-like action, and waves of contraction pass in an organized fashion from cell to cell so that material trapped in the sticky mucus layer above the cilia is moved upwards and out of the lung. This mucociliary escalator is an important part of the lung's defences. Larger bronchi also have acinar mucus-secreting glands in the submucosa which are hypertrophied in chronic bronchitis. **Alveoli** are about 0.1–0.2 mm in diameter and are lined by a thin layer of cells of which there are two types: type I pneumocytes have flattened processes which extend to cover most of the internal surface of the alveoli; type II pneumocytes are less numerous and contain lamellated structures which are concerned with the production of surfactant (Fig. 1.3). There is a potential space between the alveolar cells and the capillary basement membrane which is only apparent in disease states when it may contain fluid, fibrous tissue or a cellular infiltrate.

Alveolar ventilation

During **inspiration** the diaphragm descends, the lower ribs move upwards and outwards, and the upper ribs and sternum move upwards and forwards. The resultant expansion of the chest results in a negative intrathoracic pressure sucking air into the lungs. **Expiration** by comparison is a relatively passive procedure as the respiratory muscles gradually relax their force of contraction. About 8 litres of air are drawn into the lungs each minute at rest but not all this air reaches the alveoli. About a quarter of the air breathed in remains in the airways from the trachea to the terminal bronchioles and is not available for gas exchange. This is referred to as the **anatomical deadspace**. The distribution of air within the lungs is uneven because the resistance of the airways to airflow is not uniform and because the compliance of different parts of the lungs varies.

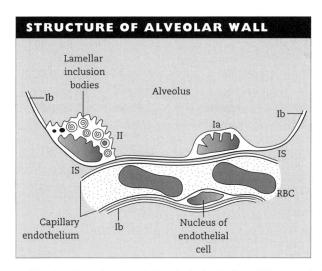

Fig. 1.3 Structure of the alveolar wall as revealed by electron microscopy. Ia, type I pneumocyte; Ib, flattened extension of type 1 pneumocyte covering most of the internal surface of the alveolus; II, type II pneumocyte with lamellar inclusion bodies which are probably the site of surfactant formation. IS, interstitial space; RBC, red blood corpuscle. Pneumocytes and endothelial cells rest upon thin continuous basement membranes which are not shown.

The greater part of total **airway resistance** to airflow during inspiration in the normal individual occurs in the larger airways — trachea, main bronchi, larynx. Increased resistance occurring in disease generally originates in the more peripheral airways. During inspiration, pulmonary elastic recoil acts as a force opening the airways. During expiration, the outward traction on the walls of the airways diminishes so that there is an increasing tendency towards closure of the airways. **Compliance** is a physiological term expressing the distensibility of the lungs. The inherent elastic properties of the lungs cause them to retract from the chest wall producing a negative intrapleural pressure. Lung compliance is expressed as *the change in lung volume brought about by unit change in transpulmonary (intrapleural) pressure*. The retractive forces of the lung are balanced by the semi-rigid structure of the thoracic cage and the action of the respiratory muscles. The effect of gravity results in the weight of the lungs keeping the upper parts under a greater stretch than the more dependent zones. The upper parts are less compliant and less receptive to air entry during inspiration. Thus, the lower zones receive more ventilation than the upper zones. Local differences in compliance and airway resistance are present to a small degree even in normal lungs but occur to a much greater extent in diseased lungs.

Lung perfusion

The lungs receive a blood supply from both the pulmonary and systemic circulations. The **pulmonary artery** arises from the right ventricle and divides into left and right pulmonary arteries, which further divide into branches accompanying the bronchial tree. The pulmonary capillary network in the alveolar walls is very dense and provides a very large surface area for gas exchange. The pulmonary venules drain laterally to the periphery of lung lobules and then pass centrally in the interlobular and intersegmental septa, ultimately joining to form the four main pulmonary veins which empty

into the left atrium. Several small **bronchial arteries** usually arise from the descending aorta and travel in the outer layers of the bronchi and bronchioles supplying the tissues of the airways down to the level of the respiratory bronchiole. Most of the blood drains into radicles of the pulmonary vein contributing a small amount of desaturated blood which accounts for part of the 'physiological shunt' observed in normal individuals. The bronchial arteries may undergo hypertrophy when there is chronic pulmonary inflammation, and major haemoptysis in diseases such as bronchiectasis or aspergilloma usually arises from the bronchial rather than the pulmonary arteries and may be treated by therapeutic bronchial artery embolization. The pulmonary circulation normally offers a much lower resistance and operates at a lower perfusion pressure than the systemic circulation. At rest in the erect position, gravity exerts a major effect on the distribution of blood with perfusion being preferentially distributed to the lung bases. Hypoxia is a potent stimulus to pulmonary vasoconstriction and seems to exert a direct effect on arterial smooth muscle. This reflex acts as a form of autoregulation, diverting blood away from underventilated areas of the lung. The pulmonary capillaries may also be compressed as they pass through the alveolar walls if alveolar pressure rises above capillary pressure.

Gas exchange and ventilation/perfusion (V/Q) relationships

During steady-state conditions the relationship between the amount of carbon dioxide produced by the body and the amount of oxygen absorbed depends upon the metabolic activity of the body and is referred to as the **respiratory quotient (RQ)**. The actual value varies from 0.7 during pure fat metabolism to 1.0 during pure carbohydrate metabolism. The RQ is usually about 0.8 but it is often assumed to be 1.0 to make calculations easier.

If carbon dioxide is being produced by the body at a constant rate the Pco_2 of alveolar air depends upon the amount of outside air that the carbon dioxide is mixed with in the alveoli, i.e. Pco_2 depends only upon alveolar ventilation and **arterial Pco_2 is a measure of alveolar ventilation**. If alveolar ventilation falls, Pco_2 rises. The level of alveolar Po_2 also varies with alveolar ventilation but measurement of arterial Po_2 is less reliable than measurement of Pco_2 as an index of alveolar ventilation because it is profoundly affected by regional changes in ventilation/perfusion ratios.

The possible combinations of Pco_2 and Po_2 are shown in Fig. 1.4. Moist atmospheric air at 37°C has a Po_2 of about 20 kPa (150 mmHg). In this model, oxygen could be exchanged with carbon dioxide in the alveoli to produce any combination of Po_2 and Pco_2 described by the oblique line which joins Po_2 20 kPa (150 mmHg) and Pco_2 20 kPa (150 mmHg). The position of the cross on this line represents the composition of a hypothetical sample of alveolar air. A fall in alveolar ventilation would result in an upward movement of this point along the line and conversely an increase in alveolar ventilation would result in a downward movement of the point. Point (a) represents the Pco_2 and Po_2 of arterial blood (it lies a little to the left of the RQ 0.8 line because of the small normal alveolar–arterial oxygen tension difference). Point (b) represents the arterial gas tension after a period of underventilation. If the arterial Pco_2 and Po_2 were those represented by point (c) this would imply that the fall in Po_2 was more than could be accounted for on the grounds of reduced alveolar ventilation.

There is normally a small difference (< 2.5 kPa or 20 mmHg) between alveolar and arterial oxygen tensions. This gradient may be roughly calculated using the simplified formula:

Alveolar–arterial $(A–a)$ gradient
$$= P_1o_2 - (Po_2 + Pco_2)$$

(P_1o_2 is the partial pressure of fractional inspired oxygen which for atmospheric air at 37°C is 20 kPa).

The quantity of gas carried by blood when exposed to different partial pressures of the

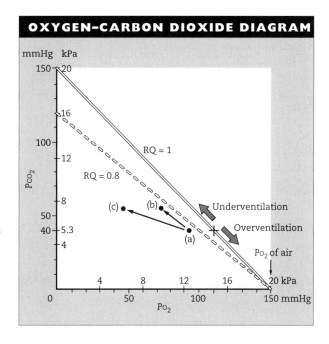

Fig. 1.4 Oxygen–carbon dioxide diagram. The continuous and interrupted lines describe the possible combinations of Pco_2 and Po_2 in alveolar air when the RQ is 1 and 0.8, respectively. (a) A hypothetical sample of arterial blood. (b) Progressive underventilation. (c) Po_2 lower than can be accounted for by underventilation alone.

OXYGEN AND CARBON DIOXIDE DISSOCIATION CURVES

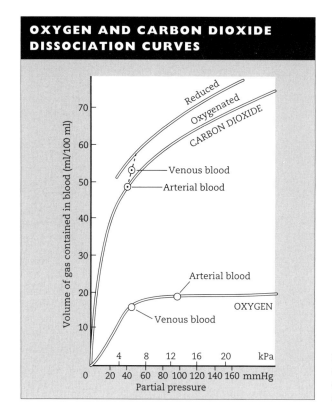

Fig. 1.5 The blood oxygen and carbon dioxide dissociation curves drawn to the same scale.

gas is described by the dissociation curve. The dissociation curves for oxygen and carbon dioxide are very different and are shown together on the same scale in Fig. 1.5. Over the range normally encountered the amount of carbon dioxide carried by the blood is roughly proportional to the $P\text{CO}_2$. However, the quantity of oxygen carried is roughly proportional to the $P\text{O}_2$ only over a very limited range of about 3–7 kPa (22–52 mmHg). Above 13.3 kPa (100 mmHg) the haemoglobin is fully saturated and hardly any additional oxygen is carried. The different shapes of the dissociation curves of oxygen and carbon dioxide explain why ventilation/perfusion mismatch has a greater effect on $P\text{O}_2$ than on $P\text{CO}_2$ levels.

Control of breathing

The **respiratory centre** in the brain stem consists of an ill-defined group of interconnected neurones, responsible for generating phasic motor discharges which ultimately pass via phrenic and intercostal nerves to the respiratory muscles. Some of the more important factors influencing the output of the respiratory centre are shown in Fig. 1.6. The $P\text{CO}_2$ of arterial blood is the most important factor in the regulation of ventilation. An **increase in $P\text{CO}_2$** stimulates sensitive areas on the surface of the brain stem directly provoking an increase in ventilation. An **increase in [H+]** (fall in pH) also stimulates ventilation. **Hypoxaemia** sensitizes the respiratory centre to carbon dioxide probably via an effect on the carotid and aortic bodies. However, the effect of hypoxaemia is small above a $P\text{O}_2$ of about 8.8 kPa (60 mmHg). Input from **higher centres** is important, with alarm and excitement stimulating ventilation, and sleep and coma reducing the response to normal ventilatory stimuli. The

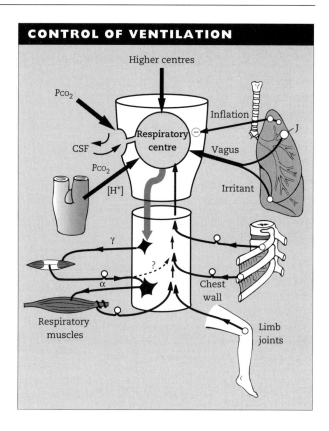

CONTROL OF VENTILATION

Fig. 1.6 Control of ventilation: some of the more important factors involved (see text).

vagus nerve carries afferent stimuli from the respiratory tract which may influence breathing. In animals, stretching of the lungs causes reflex inhibition of subsequent inspiration (Hering–Breuer inflation reflex) although the importance of this reflex is doubtful in humans. Stimulation of **J receptors**, situated deep in the lung parenchyma, increases ventilation. Excitation of stretch receptors in muscles, joints, and chest wall may also enhance ventilation.

Further reading

Brewis RAL, White FE. Anatomy of the thorax. In: Brewis RAL, Corrin B, Geddes DM, Gibson GJ, eds. *Respiratory Medicine.* London: WB Saunders Co., 1995: 22–53.

Cotes JE. *Lung Function: Assessment and Application in Medicine.* Oxford: Blackwell Science, 1993.

Gibson GJ. *Clinical Tests of Respiratory Function.* Oxford: Chapman and Hall, 1996.

West JB. *Pulmonary Pathophysiology — The Essentials.* Baltimore: Williams and Wilkins, 1987.

CHAPTER 2

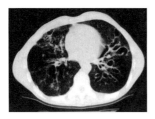

Symptoms and Signs of Respiratory Disease

History taking

History taking is of paramount importance in the assessment of a patient with respiratory disease. Do not be tempted to proceed to complex investigations without having taken a detailed history. Difficult diagnostic problems are more often solved by a carefully taken history than by laboratory tests. It is during history taking that the doctor also gets to know the patient and the patient's fears and concerns. The relationship of trust thus established forms the basis of the therapeutic partnership. Start by asking the patient to describe the symptoms in his or her own words. Listening to the patient's account of the symptoms is an active process in which the doctor is seeking clues to underlying processes, judging which items require further exploration and noting the patient's attitude and anxieties. By carefully posed questions the skilled clinician directs the patient to focus on pertinent points, to clarify crucial details and to explore areas of possible importance. History-taking skills develop with experience and with a greater knowledge of respiratory disease.

Symptoms (Table 2.1)

Dyspnoea

This is an unpleasant sensation of **being unable to breathe easily**, i.e. breathlessness. Analysis of this symptom requires an assessment of the speed of onset, progression, periodicity and precipitating and relieving factors. The severity of dyspnoea is graded according to the patient's exercise tolerance, e.g. dyspnoeic on climbing a flight of stairs; dyspnoeic at rest. Onset may be sudden as in the case of a pneumothorax, or gradual and progressive as in chronic obstructive pulmonary disease (COPD). An episodic dyspnoea pattern is characteristic of asthma with symptoms typically being precipitated by cold air or exercise. **Orthopnoea** is dyspnoea which occurs when lying flat and is relieved by sitting upright. It is a characteristic feature of pulmonary oedema or diaphragm paralysis but is found also in many respiratory diseases. **Paroxysmal nocturnal dyspnoea** (PND) refers to the phenomenon of the patient waking up breathless at night. It is most commonly associated with pulmonary oedema but must be distinguished from the nocturnal wheeze and the sleep disturbance of asthma. It is important to note what words the patient uses to describe the symptoms: 'tightness in the chest' may indicate breathlessness or angina. Dyspnoea is not a symptom which is specific to respiratory disease and it may be associated with various cardiac diseases, anxiety, anaemia and metabolic states such as ketoacidosis.

Wheeze

This is a whistling or sighing noise which is characteristic of air passing through a narrow tube. The sound of wheeze can be mimicked by

RESPIRATORY SYMPTOMS
Dyspnoea
Wheeze
Cough
Sputum
Haemoptysis
Chest pain

Table 2.1 Main respiratory symptoms.

breathing out almost to residual volume and then giving a further sharp forced expiration. Wheeze is a characteristic feature of airways obstruction caused by asthma or COPD but can also occur in pulmonary oedema. In asthma, wheeze is characteristically worse on waking in the morning and may be precipitated by exercise or cold air. Wheeze which improves at weekends or on holidays away from work and deteriorates on return to the work environment is suggestive of occupational asthma. In asthma and COPD wheezing is more prominent in expiration. An inspiratory wheeze—**stridor**—is a feature of disease of the central airways, e.g. obstruction of the trachea by a carcinoma.

Cough and sputum

Cough is a forceful expiratory blast produced by contraction of the abdominal muscles with bracing by the intercostal muscles and sudden opening of the glottis. It is a protective reflex which removes secretions or inhaled solid material, and it is provoked by physical or chemical stimulation of irritant receptors in the larynx, trachea or bronchial tree. Cough may be dry or associated with sputum production. The duration and nature of the cough should be assessed, and precipitating and relieving factors explored. It is important to examine any **sputum** produced, noting whether it is mucoid, purulent or blood-stained, for example. Cough occurring on exercise or disturbing sleep at night is a feature of asthma. A transient cough productive of purulent sputum is very common in respiratory tract infections. A weak ineffective cough which fails to clear secretions from the airways is a feature of bulbar palsy or expiratory muscle weakness, and predisposes the patient to aspiration pneumonia. Cough is often triggered by the accumulation of sputum in the respiratory tract. Chronic bronchitis is defined as cough productive of sputum on most days for at least 3 months of 2 consecutive years. Bronchiectasis is characterized by the production of copious amounts of purulent sputum. A chronic cough may also be caused by gastro-oesophageal reflux with aspiration, sinusitis with post-nasal drip, and occasionally by drugs (e.g. captopril). Violent coughing can generate sufficient force to produce a '**cough fracture**' of a rib or to impede venous return and cerebral perfusion causing '**cough syncope**'. Patients with alveolar cell carcinoma sometimes produce very large volumes of watery sputum: **bronchorrhoea**. Patients with coal-worker's pneumoconiosis will occasionally cough up black material: **melanoptysis**.

Haemoptysis

This is the **coughing up of blood**. It is a very important symptom which requires investigation. In particular, it may be the first clue to the presence of bronchial carcinoma, and early investigation may detect the tumour at a stage when curative surgery can be performed. All patients with haemoptysis should have a chest X-ray performed, and further investigations such as bronchoscopy, computed tomography (CT), sputum cytology and microbiology may be indicated depending on the circumstances. The most important causes of haemoptysis are bronchial carcinoma, lung infections (pneumonia, bronchiectasis, tuberculosis), chronic bronchitis, pulmonary infarction, pulmonary oedema and pulmonary vasculitis (Table 2.2). In some cases no cause is found and the origin of the blood may have been in the upper airway, e.g. nose (epistaxis), pharynx or gums.

Chest pain

Pain which is aggravated by inspiration or coughing is described as **pleuritic pain**, and

CAUSES OF HAEMOPTYSIS

Tumours
Bronchial carcinoma
Laryngeal carcinoma

Infections
Tuberculosis
Pneumonia
Bronchiectasis
Infective bronchitis

Infarction
Pulmonary embolism

Pulmonary oedema
Left ventricular failure
Mitral stenosis

Pulmonary vasculitis
Goodpasture's syndrome
Wegener's granulomatosis

Table 2.2 Major causes of haemoptysis.

the patient can often be seen to wince when breathing in, as the pain 'catches'. Irritation of the pleura may result from inflammation (pleurisy), infection (pneumonia), infarction of underlying lung (pulmonary embolism) or tumour (malignant pleural effusion). Chest wall pain resulting from injury to the intercostal muscles or fractured ribs, for example, is also aggravated by inspiration or coughing and is associated with tenderness at the point of injury.

In addition to these major respiratory symptoms it is important to consider other associated symptoms. For example, **anorexia** and **weight loss** are features of malignancy or chronic lung infections (e.g. lung abscess). **Pyrexia** and **sweating** are features of acute (e.g. pneumonia) and chronic infections (e.g. tuberculosis). **Lethargy**, malaise and confusion may be features of hypoxaemia. **Headaches**, particularly on awakening in the morning, may be a symptom of hypercapnia. **Oedema** may indicate cor pulmonale. **Snor-** ing and daytime **somnolence** may indicate obstructive sleep apnoea syndrome. **Hoarseness** of the voice may indicate damage to the recurrent laryngeal nerve by a tumour.

Many respiratory diseases have their roots in previous **childhood lung disease** or in the **patient's environment** so that it is crucial to make specific enquiries concerning these points during history taking.

History

Past medical history

Did the patient suffer any major illness in childhood? Did the patient have frequent absences from school? Was the patient able to play games at school? Did any abnormalities declare themselves at a pre-employment medical examination or on chest X-ray? Has the patient ever been admitted to hospital with chest disease? A long history of childhood 'bronchitis' may in fact indicate asthma. Severe whooping cough or measles in childhood may cause bronchiectasis. Tuberculosis acquired early in life may re-activate many years later.

General medical history

Has the patient any systemic illness which may involve the lungs, e.g. rheumatoid arthritis? Is the patient taking any medications which might affect the lungs, e.g. amiodarone, which can cause interstitial lung disease, or β-blockers (e.g. atenolol), which may provoke bronchospasm? What effect will the patient's lung disease have on other illnesses, e.g. fitness for surgery?

Family history

Is there any history of lung disease in the family? An increased prevalence of lung disease in a family may result from 'shared genes', i.e. inherited traits such as cystic fibrosis, α_1-antitrypsin deficiency, asthmatic tendency; or from 'shared environment', e.g. tuberculosis.

Social history

Does the patient smoke, or has he or she ever

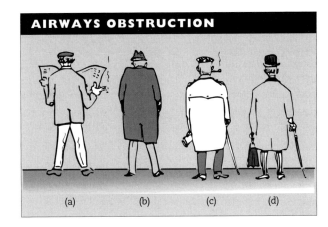

AIRWAYS OBSTRUCTION

(a)   (b)   (c)   (d)

Fig. 2.1 Which man has airways obstruction? (Answer at foot of p. 12.)

smoked? Is the patient exposed to passive smoking at home? It is important to obtain a clear account of total smoking exposure over the years so as to assess the patient's risk for diseases such as lung cancer or COPD. Does the patient keep any pets or participate in any sports (e.g. diving) or hobbies (e.g. pigeon racing) which may be important in assessing the lung disease?

Occupational history

What occupations has the patient had over the years, what tasks were performed and what materials used? Did symptoms show a direct relationship to the work environment as in the case of occupational asthma improving away from work and deteriorating on return to work? Has the patient been exposed to substances which may give rise to disease many years later as in the case of mesothelioma arising from exposure to asbestos 20–40 years previously?

Examination

Examination of the respiratory system is, of course, integrated into the general examination of the patient as a whole, but outlining the different stages in the assessment of the respiratory system is useful in focusing attention on the features of particular importance to be

sought. Powers of observation are developed by training, and knowing what to look for and how to look for it are learned by experience.

General examination

Be alert to clues to respiratory disease which may be evident from the moment the patient is first seen (Fig. 2.1) or which become apparent during history taking. These include the rate and **character of breathing**, signs of respiratory distress such as **use of accessory muscles** of respiration (e.g. sternocleidomastoids), the **shape of the chest**, spine and shoulders, and the character of any **cough**. **Hoarseness** of the voice may be a clue to recurrent laryngeal nerve damage by a carcinoma. **Stridor** or **wheeze** may be audible. Count the **respiratory rate** over a period of 30 seconds. Avoid proceeding directly to examination of the chest but first pause to look for signs in the hands such as **clubbing, nicotine staining** or **features of rheumatoid arthritis**. Signs of carbon dioxide retention include peripheral **vasodilatation** and **asterixis**, a flapping tremor detected by asking the patient to spread his or her fingers and cock the wrists back. It may be accentuated by applying gentle pressure against the patient's hands in this position. Count the **pulse rate** over 30 seconds and note any abnormalities in rhythm (e.g. atrial fibrillation) or character (e.g. a bounding pulse of carbon dioxide retention).

Next examine the head and neck, particularly seeking signs of **cyanosis**, **anaemia** (pallor of conjunctiva), elevation of **jugular venous pressure** or **lymph node enlargement**. Be alert for uncommon signs such as **Horner's syndrome** (ptosis, meiosis, enophthalmos, anhydrosis) indicating damage to the sympathetic nerves by a tumour situated at the lung apex (see Chapter 13).

Clubbing

This is increased curvature of the nail with loss of the angle between the nail and nail bed (Fig. 2.2). It is a very important sign which is associated with a number of diseases (Table 2.3), most notably bronchial carcinoma and fibrotic lung disease, such as cryptogenic fibrosing alveolitis and asbestosis. Advanced clubbing is sometimes associated with hypertrophic pulmonary osteoarthropathy in which there is new bone formation in the subperiosteal region of the long bones of the arms and legs which is detectable on X-ray and is associated with pain and tenderness.

Cyanosis

This is a bluish discolouration of the skin and mucous membranes due to an excessive amount of reduced haemoglobin (usually >5 g/dl). **Central cyanosis** is best seen on the tip of the tongue and is the cardinal sign of hypoxaemia, although it is not a sensitive sign since it is not usually detectable until the oxygen saturation has fallen to well below 90%, corresponding to a Po_2 of <8 kPa (60 mmHg). Cyanosis is more difficult to detect if the

CLUBBING

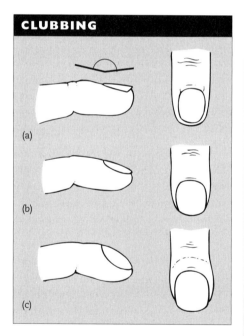

Fig. 2.2 Clubbing. (a) Normal, showing the 'angle'. (b) Early clubbing; the angle is absent. (c) Advanced clubbing. The nail shows increased curvature in all directions, the angle is absent, the base of the nail is raised up by spongy tissue and the end of the digit is expanded.

CAUSES OF CLUBBING

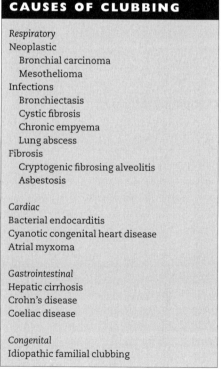

Respiratory
Neoplastic
  Bronchial carcinoma
  Mesothelioma
Infections
  Bronchiectasis
  Cystic fibrosis
  Chronic empyema
  Lung abscess
Fibrosis
  Cryptogenic fibrosing alveolitis
  Asbestosis

Cardiac
Bacterial endocarditis
Cyanotic congenital heart disease
Atrial myxoma

Gastrointestinal
Hepatic cirrhosis
Crohn's disease
Coeliac disease

Congenital
Idiopathic familial clubbing

Table 2.3 Causes of clubbing.

Answer to question in Fig. 2.1: (b) has airways obstruction—note the high position of the shoulders.

patient is anaemic or has dark-coloured skin. Because of the poor sensitivity of cyanosis it is essential to measure oxygenation by oximetry or arterial blood gas sampling in patients at risk for hypoxaemia. **Peripheral cyanosis** may be caused by local circulatory slowing in the peripheries resulting in more complete extraction of oxygen from the blood, e.g. blue hands and ears in cold weather.

Jugular veins

Jugular veins are examined with the patient in a semi-reclining position with the trunk at an angle of about 45° from the horizontal. The head is turned slightly to the opposite side and fully supported so that the sternocleidomastoid muscles are relaxed. The jugular venous pulse is seen as a diffuse superficial pulsation of multiple wave form which is distinct from the carotid arterial pulse. The height of the pulse wave is measured from the top of the oscillating column of blood vertically to the sternal angle. The jugular venous pressure normally falls during inspiration. It is elevated in right heart failure which may occur as a result of pulmonary embolism or cor pulmonale in COPD, for example. Other signs of right heart failure such as hepatomegaly and peripheral oedema may also be present.

Chest examination

Ask the patient to undress to the waist, and proceed to examine the chest in a methodical way using the techniques of inspection, palpation, percussion and auscultation.

Inspection

Look at the chest from the front, back and sides noting the overall **shape** and any **asymmetry**, **scars** or **skeletal abnormality**. The normal chest is flattened anteroposteriorly whereas the hyperinflated chest of COPD is barrel shaped with an increased anteroposterior diameter. Watch the **movement** of the chest carefully as the patient breathes in and out. Diminished movement of one side of the chest is a clue to disease on that side. Overall movement is reduced if the lungs are hyper-inflated (e.g. emphysema) or have reduced compliance (e.g. fibrosis). The costal margins normally move upwards and outwards in inspiration as the chest expands. In a chest which is already severely overinflated (e.g. COPD) there is sometimes paradoxical movement of the costal margins such that they are drawn inwards during inspiration: **costal margin paradox** (Fig. 2.3). The abdominal wall normally moves outwards on inspiration as the diaphragm descends. **Abdominal paradox**, in which the abdominal wall moves inwards during inspiration when the patient is supine, is a sign of diaphragm weakness.

Palpation

Chest movements during respiration may be more easily appreciated by placing the hands exactly symmetrically on either side of the upper sternum with the thumbs in the midline. The relative movement of the two hands and the separation of the thumbs reflect the overall movement of the chest and any asymmetry between the two sides. The position of the mediastinum is assessed by locating the **tracheal position** and the cardiac **apex beat**. Inserting a finger between the trachea and the sternocleidomastoid muscle on each side is a useful way of detecting any tracheal deviation. Running a finger gently up and down the trachea from the cricoid cartilage to the sternal notch may indicate the direction of the trachea as it enters the chest. Reduction in the **crico-sternal distance** is a sign of a hyperinflated chest. The apex beat is the most inferior and lateral point at which the cardiac impulse can be felt. The intercostal space in which the apex beat is felt should be counted down from the second intercostal space which is just below the sternal angle, and its location should also be related to landmarks such as the mid-clavicular or anterior axillary lines. It is normally located in the fifth left intercostal space in the mid-clavicular line. The mediastinum may be deviated towards or away from the side of disease. For example, fibrosis of the apex of the lung caused by previous tuberculosis may *pull* the trachea to that side, whereas a

MOVEMENT OF THE COSTAL MARGIN

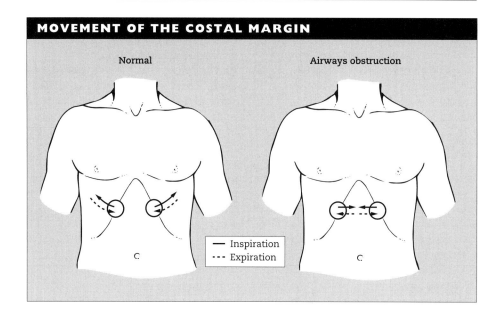

Normal   Airways obstruction

— Inspiration
--- Expiration

Fig. 2.3 Movement of the costal margin. The arrows indicate the direction of movement in normal individuals and in those with airways obstruction (see text).

large pleural effusion or tension pneumothorax may *push* the trachea and apex beat away from the side of the lesion. **Tactile fremitus** refers to the ability to palpate vibrations set up by the voice in the large airways and transmitted to the chest wall. Ask the patient to say 'ninety-nine' or 'one, one, one' and palpate the vibrations, which are reduced in conditions such as pleural effusion or pleural thickening since they muffle the transmission of the vibrations from the lung to the chest wall (Fig. 2.4). Consolidation of the lung may sometimes enhance transmission of the vibration.

Percussion

Percussion over normal air-filled lung produces a **resonant note** whereas percussion over solid organs such as the liver or heart produces a **dull note**. Abnormal dullness is found over areas of lung consolidation (e.g. lobar pneumonia) or fluid (e.g. pleural effusion). **Hyper-**resonance may be present in emphysema or over the area of a pneumothorax, although it is rarely a reliable sign. Percussion technique is important and requires practice. The resting finger should be placed flat against the chest wall in an intercostal space. The percussing finger should strike the dorsal surface of the middle phalanx and should be lifted clear after each percussion stroke. All areas should be percussed, paying particular attention to comparison between the two sides. When percussing the back of the chest it is helpful to ask the patient to rotate his or her arms such that one elbow is placed on top of the other in order to bring the scapulae forward and out of the way.

Auscultation

Listen with the diaphragm or bell of the stethoscope to the **intensity** and **character** of the **breath sounds**, comparing both sides symmetrically, and note any **added sounds** (e.g. wheeze, crackles, pleural rub). The sources of audible sound in the lungs are turbulent airflow in the larynx and central airways and the voice. Reduction in the intensity of breath sounds (sometimes loosely referred to as reduced 'air

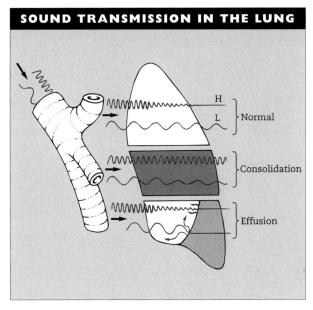

Fig. 2.4 Summary of sound transmission in the lung. Sound is generated either by turbulence in the larynx and large airways, or by the voice. Both sources are a mixture of high- (H) and low- (L) pitched components. *Normal aerated lung* filters off the high-pitched component but transmits the low-pitched component quite well. This results in soft low-pitched breath sounds, well-conducted vocal resonance and easily palpable very-low-pitched sound (vocal fremitus). *Consolidated lung* transmits high-pitched sound well and filters off some of the lower pitched sound. This results in loud high-pitched breath sounds (bronchial breathing), high-pitched bleating vocal resonance (aegophony) and easy transmission of high-pitched consonants of speech (whispering pectoriloquy). *Pleural effusion* causes reduction in the transmission of all sound — probably because of reflection of sound waves at the air–fluid interface. Breath sounds are absent, vocal resonance much reduced and vocal fremitus is absent.

entry') over an area of lung is an important sign which may, for example, indicate obstruction of a large bronchus preventing air from entering a lobe of the lung, or the presence of a pleural effusion reducing transmission of sound to the stethoscope. In normal individuals the **inspiratory phase** of respiration is usually longer than the **expiratory phase**. Prolongation of the expiratory phase is a feature of airways obstruction and this is often accompanied by **wheeze (rhonchi)** — a high-pitched whistling or sighing sound. Diffuse wheeze is a feature of asthma or COPD. Wheeze localized to one side, or one area of the lung, suggests obstruction of a bronchus by a carcinoma or foreign body (e.g. inhaled peanut). **Crackles (crepitations)** may be loud and coarse or fine and high pitched, and may occur early or late in inspiration. It is thought that crackles are produced by the opening of previously closed bronchioles. The 'crackling' noise may be imitated by rolling a few hairs together close to the ear. Early crackles are sometimes heard at the beginning of inspiration in patients with COPD but these usually disappear when the patient is asked to cough. Persistent pan-inspiratory or late-inspiratory crackles are a feature of pulmonary oedema, lung fibrosis (e.g. cryptogenic fibrosing alveolitis) or bronchiectasis. During inspiration, areas of lung open up in sequence according to their compliance (distensibility). In airways

SIGNS OF LOCALIZED LUNG DISEASE

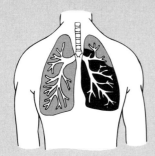

Consolidation (e.g. lobar pneumonia)

- Movement of affected side may be reduced
- Percussion note is dull
- Crackles may be heard
- Bronchial breathing may be present
- Whispering pectoriloquy and aegophony may occur
- Vocal fremitus and resonance are sometimes increased

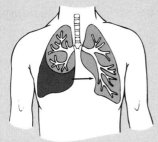

Pleural effusion

- Trachea and apex beat may be displaced away from the effusion if it is large
- Movement of affected side may be reduced
- Percussion note is stony dull
- Vocal fremitus and resonance are reduced
- Breath sounds are reduced

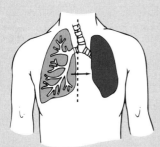

Collapsed lung (atelectasis)

- Trachea and apex beat may be displaced to the side of collapse
- Movement of affected side is reduced
- Breath sounds are diminished

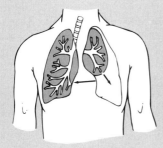

Tension pneumothorax

- Trachea and apex beat are displaced away from the affected side
- Percussion note may be hyper-resonant
- Breath sounds are reduced over pneumothorax
- Vocal fremitus and resonance may be reduced

Fig. 2.5 Signs of localized lung disease.

obstruction there may be terminal airway closure during expiration particularly in relatively compliant (floppy) parts of the lung damaged by emphysema. During inspiration air initially enters these areas more readily and crackles are probably produced by the opening of these airways early in inspiration. Coarse late inspiratory crackles are particularly associated with diseases where there is reduced lung compliance (increased stiffness) which is to some extent patchily distributed. During inspiration, air first enters the more compliant parts of the lung and then enters the stiffer parts later in inspiration as elastic recoil forces build up in the stretching lung. **Pleural rubs** are 'creaking' sounds which are often quite localized and indicate roughening of the normally slippery pleural surfaces.

Vocal resonance is assessed by listening over the chest with the stethoscope as the patient says 'ninety-nine' or 'one, one, one' in much the same way as vocal fremitus is palpated. Normal aerated lung transmits the booming low-pitched components of speech and attenuates the high frequencies. Consolidated lung, however, filters off the low frequencies and transmits the higher frequencies so that speech takes on a bleating quality, aegophony. The facilitated transmission of high frequencies can be demonstrated by the clear transmission of whispering over consolidated lung, **whispering pectoriloquy**. The term '**bronchial breathing**' refers to the harsher breath sounds normally heard over the trachea and main bronchi. It is also heard over areas of consolidated lung which conduct the higher frequency 'hiss' component from the larger airways.

Signs

See Fig. 2.5 for signs of localized lung disease. It is important to realize that major disease of the lungs may be present without any detectable physical signs and it is therefore essential to obtain a chest X-ray where there is good reason to suspect localized lung disease.

Further reading

Naish JM, Read AE, Burns-Cox CJ. *The Clinical Apprentice*. Bristol: John Wright and Sons, 1978.
Ogilvie C. *Chamberlain's Symptoms and Signs in Clinical Medicine*. Bristol: John Wright and Sons, 1980.

CHAPTER 3

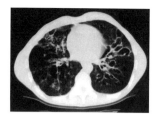

Pulmonary Function Tests

Introduction

Pulmonary function tests are useful in **defining** respiratory disorders, in **quantifying** the severity of any deficit and in **monitoring** the course of the disease. Simple tests such as spirometry or measurement of peak expiratory flow (PEF) may be performed **in the consulting room, at the bedside** or by the patients themselves **at home**, whereas more complex tests require the facilities of a **lung function laboratory**. Normal values depend on the patient's height, age and sex, and tables and prediction equations are available for determining a patient's predicted normal value.

The patient's test result may be compared with the mean reference value and standard deviation of results obtained in the healthy population or expressed as a percentage of the population's mean reference value. Pulmonary function tests should not be interpreted in isolation and should be considered in the context of all additional information concerning the patient.

Lung volumes (Fig. 3.1)

Tidal volume is the volume of air which enters and leaves the lungs during normal

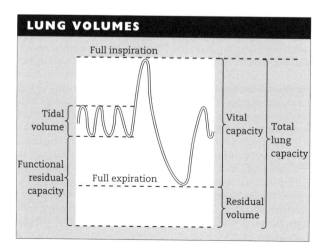

LUNG VOLUMES

Full inspiration

Tidal volume

Functional residual capacity

Full expiration

Vital capacity

Total lung capacity

Residual volume

Fig. 3.1 Total lung capacity and its subdivisions.

breathing. The volume of gas within the lungs at the end of a normal expiration is the **functional residual capacity**. The volume of gas in the lungs after a full inspiration is the **total lung capacity**. After a full expiration there is still some gas remaining in the lungs: the **residual volume**. **Vital capacity** (VC) is the volume of air expelled by a maximum expiration from a position of full inspiration. VC and its subdivisions can be measured directly by spirometry whereas measurements of residual volume and total lung capacity require the use of gas dilution or plethysmography methods.

Spirometry

Spirometry measures changes in lung volume by recording changes in the volume of air exchanged through the airway opening (Fig. 3.2). Because residual volume cannot be exhaled, spirometry measurements are limited to VC and its subdivisions. One of the most useful techniques is to plot the volume of air exhaled from a patient's lungs against time

during a forced expiratory manoeuvre: the **forced expiratory spirogram** (see Fig. 3.4, p. 22).

Vital capacity

Vital capacity is the **volume of air expelled by a maximum expiration from a position of full inspiration**. It is often derived from a forced expiratory spirogram, with the patient exhaling with maximum effort, in which case it is referred to as the **forced vital capacity** (FVC). It may also be measured by a slow exhalation and this is sometimes referred to as the **'slow'** VC. In normal individuals, slow VC and FVC are very similar but in patients with airways obstruction air trapping occurs during forced expiration so that the FVC may be significantly smaller than the slow VC. The following circumstances may reduce VC:
• reduced lung compliance (e.g. lung fibrosis, loss of lung volume);
• chest deformity (e.g. kyphoscoliosis, ankylosing spondylitis);
• muscle weakness (e.g. myopathy, myasthenia gravis);
• airways obstruction (e.g. chronic obstructive

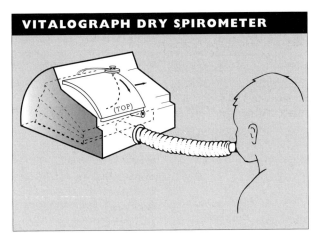

VITALOGRAPH DRY SPIROMETER

(TOP)

Fig. 3.2 Schematic view of Vitalograph dry spirometer. The main components are a bellows and a moving record chart. An arm attached to the bellows carries a writing point which moves across the chart as air enters the bellows. As soon as the bellows moves, a microswitch is triggered and a motor causes the record chart to move steadily from left to right. The combination of lateral movement of the chart and forward movement of the writing point causes an oblique line to be inscribed upon the chart (see Fig. 3.4).

pulmonary disease (COPD) — air trapping causes increased residual volume and reduced VC).

Forced expiratory volume in 1 second

Forced expiratory volume in 1 second (FEV_1) is the **volume of air expelled in the first second of a maximal forced expiration from a position of full inspiration**. It is reduced in any condition that reduces VC but it is particularly reduced when there is **diffuse airways obstruction**.

Forced expiratory volume in 1 second/forced vital capacity ratio

Normally, during a forced expiratory manoeuvre at least 75% of the air is expelled in the first second. In diffuse airways obstruction the FEV_1 is affected to a greater extent than the FVC and the ratio of FEV_1/FVC is reduced to below 0.75. This pattern is referred to as an **obstructive defect**. When lung volume is restricted by pulmonary fibrosis or rigidity of the chest wall for example, the VC is reduced and the FEV_1 is also reduced in proportion so that the FEV_1/FVC ratio is normal. This pattern of ventilatory impairment is referred to as a **restrictive defect**.

Maximal mid-expiratory flow

In addition to FEV_1 and FVC a number of other indices may be calculated from a forced expiratory spirogram. The maximal mid-expiratory flow **measured over the middle half of forced expiration** ($FEF_{25-75\%}$) reflects changes in the smaller **peripheral airways** whereas PEF and FEV_1 are predominantly influenced by diffuse changes of the medium-sized and larger airways.

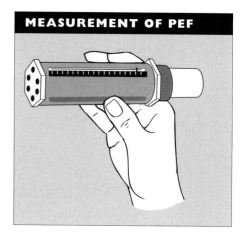

Fig. 3.3 Measurement of peak expiratory flow (PEF). The Wright Mini Peak Flow Meter. The subject takes a *full inspiration*, applies the lips to the mouthpiece and makes a sudden maximal expiratory blast. A piston is pushed down the inside of the cylinder progressively exposing a slot in the top, until a position of rest is reached. The position of the piston is indicated by a marker and PEF read from a scale. It is customary to take the best of three properly performed attempts as the PEF.

dependent on effort but is mainly determined by the calibre of the airways and is therefore an index of **diffuse airways obstruction**. It is particularly useful in monitoring the course of asthma (see Chapter 11).

Flow–volume loop

The familiar spirometer trace plots volume against time (Fig. 3.4). Forced ventilatory manoeuvres may also be displayed by plotting **flow against volume in both expiration and inspiration**. This may be done using a pneumotachograph, which is a transducer comprising a small resistance to airflow through which the patient breathes. Pressure drop across this resistance is proportional to airflow. The pressure is converted to an electrical signal and displayed on an oscilloscope or plotter. The volume of air moved can be

Peak expiratory flow

PEF is the **maximum rate of airflow** which can be achieved **during a sudden forced expiration** from a position of full inspiration (Fig. 3.3). The best of three attempts is usually accepted as the peak flow rate. It is somewhat derived from electrical integration of the flow signal. A normal flow–volume loop is shown in Fig. 3.5. PEF is reached early in expiration from total lung capacity and is faster than peak inspiratory flow. There is a steady fall in expiratory flow as expiration progresses. The flow–volume loop is particularly used in assessing localized narrowing of the central airways as illustrated in Figs 3.6 and 3.7. Interpretation of the flow–volume loop may be difficult and the inspiratory portion is less reproducible than the expiratory portion, but flow–volume loops are useful in suggesting less common causes of **central airways obstruction** such as bilateral vocal cord palsy, tracheal tumours or tracheal compression by mediastinal disease. In practice, there is often difficulty in diagnosing these conditions, usually because the possibility is not considered and the patient is misdiagnosed as having asthma. Flow–volume loops or subtle changes on spirometry may point to the diagnosis and indicate the need for a definitive investigation such as bronchoscopy or computed tomography, for example.

Total lung capacity

Whereas VC and its subdivisions can be measured directly by spirometry, measurement of residual volume and total lung capacity require the use of **helium dilution** or **plethysmography** methods. In the dilution technique a gas of known helium concentration is breathed through a closed circuit and the volume of gas in the lungs is calculated from a measure of the dilution of the helium, which, being an inert gas, is neither absorbed nor metabolized. This dilution method measures only gas in communication with the airways and tends to underestimate total lung capacity in patients with severe airways obstruction because of the presence of poorly ventilating bullae. The body plethysmograph is a large airtight box that allows the simultaneous determination of pressure–volume relationships in the thorax of a patient placed inside the box. When the

plethysmograph is sealed, changes in lung volume are reflected by an increase in pressure within the plethysmograph. Plethysmography tends to overestimate total lung capacity because it measures all intrathoracic gas, including gas in bullae, cysts, stomach and oesophagus. The **chest X-ray** can be used to give a rough estimate of total lung capacity. In airways disease, residual volume is often increased as a manifestation of air trapping and total lung capacity increased as a manifestation of hyperinflation. Total lung capacity is reduced in restrictive lung disease.

Transfer factor for carbon monoxide

The **rate at which gas passes from the alveoli to the blood stream** can be measured using a low concentration of carbon monoxide. The transfer of carbon monoxide across the alveolar capillary membrane is similar to that of oxygen. Oxygen diffusion is difficult to measure because transport stops when haemoglobin becomes saturated. At one time it was thought that the main factor limiting gas exchange in disease was the ability of gases to diffuse across the alveolar capillary membrane. This led to the concept of **diffusing capacity** for carbon monoxide ($D_L co$). It was later realized that many other factors (e.g. ventilation/perfusion matching) influenced gas transfer and the expression was renamed **transfer factor** ($T_L co$). The **transfer coefficient** ($K co$) is an expression of gas transfer standardized for the alveolar volume (V_A).

Single-breath method (Fig. 3.8)
The patient inspires a gas mixture of helium and carbon monoxide, holds the breath for 10 seconds and then breathes out. An initial volume equivalent to the deadspace is discarded and then a sample of the expired gas is collected and analysed for alveolar concentrations of helium and carbon monoxide. The change in concentration of helium between the

FORCED EXPIRATORY SPIROGRAM TRACINGS

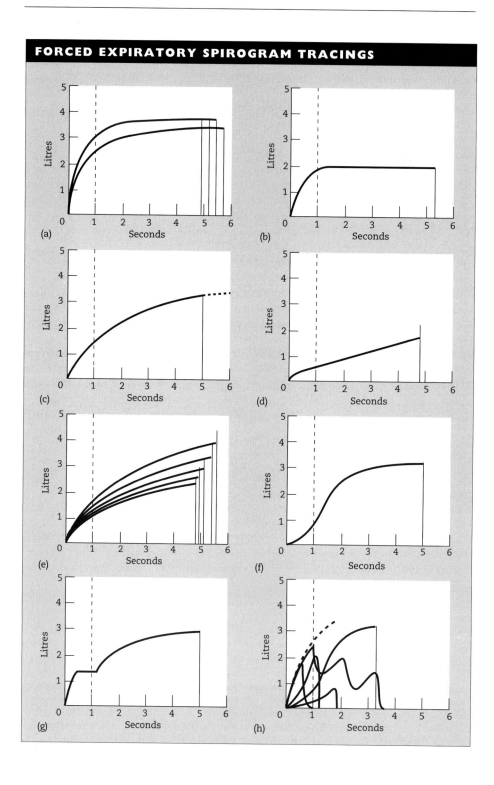

inspired and alveolar sample is the result of gas dilution and gives a measurement of the alveolar gas volume (V_A). The expired concentration of carbon monoxide is also lower than the inspired level but the fall is proportionately greater than in the case of helium because some of the carbon monoxide has been absorbed into the blood stream. The rate of uptake of carbon monoxide can then be calculated as the uptake of carbon monoxide per minute per unit of partial pressure of carbon monoxide (mmol/min/kPa), or as the carbon monoxide transfer coefficient (Kco) which is the $T_L$co standardized for V_A.

Steady-state method

The patient breathes air containing a known low concentration of carbon monoxide from a Douglas bag and expired air is collected in another Douglas bag over a timed period of some minutes. The rate of carbon monoxide transfer can be calculated from the difference between inspired and expired concentrations. A mean alveolar carbon monoxide level can be calculated by estimating a deadspace ventilation for carbon dioxide and assuming that this same volume was filled with unchanged inspired carbon monoxide mixture. The shortfall in expired carbon monoxide must then be

---

Fig. 3.4 Forced expiratory spirogram tracing obtained with a Vitalograph spirometer.
(a) *Normal.* Four expirations have been made. Three of these were true maximal forced expirations as indicated by their *reproducibility.* The forced expiratory volume in 1 second (FEV_1) is 3.2 litres and the forced vital capacity (FVC) is 3.8 litres. The forced expiratory ratio (FEV_1/FVC) is 84%.
(b) *Restrictive ventilatory defect.* Patient with pulmonary fibrosis. The FVC in this case was 2 litres less than the predicted value for the subject. The FEV_1 is also reduced below the predicted value but it represents a large part of the FVC. The forced expiratory ratio is greater than 90%.
(c) *Obstructive ventilatory defect.* The FEV_1 is much reduced. The rate of airflow is severely reduced as indicated by the reduced slope of the curve. Note that the forced expiratory time is increased—the patient is still blowing out at 5 seconds. The vital capacity has not been adequately recorded in this case because the patient did not continue the expiration after the chart stopped moving; he or she could have expired further. (This is a common technical error.)
(d) *Severe airways obstruction.* The FEV_1 is about 0.5 litres. FVC is also reduced but not so strikingly as FEV_1. Forced expiratory ratio 23%. Very low expiratory flow rate. This pattern of a very brief initial rapid phase followed by a straight line indicating little change in maximal flow rate with change in lung volume is sometimes associated with severe emphysema.
(e) *Airways obstruction and bronchial hyperreactivity.*

Five expirations have been made. FEV_1 and FVC become lower with each expiration. Patient with asthma. These features suggest poor control of asthma and liability to severe attacks.
(f) *A non-maximal expiration.* Compare with (a). In a true forced expiration the steepest part of the curve always occurs at the beginning of expiration which is not the case in (f). A falsely low FEV_1 and forced expiratory ratio are obtained. Usually the patient has not understood what is required or is unable to coordinate his or her actions. Some patients wish to appear worse than they really are. This pattern is unlikely to be mistaken for a true forced expiration because of its shape and because it cannot be reproduced repeatedly.
(g) *Escape of air* from the nose or lips during expiration.
(h) *Inability to perform the manoeuvre.* Five attempts have been made. In some the patient has breathed in and out. Other attempts are either not maximal forced expirations or are unfinished. Bizarre patterns such as this are often seen in patients with psychogenic breathlessness and in the elderly and demented. Even with poor cooperation it is often possible to obtain useful information. In the example shown (h), significant airways obstruction can be excluded because of the steep slope of at least two of the expirations which follow an identical course and show appropriate curvature (dotted line) and the FVC can be estimated as not less than 3.2 litres. The pattern seen in large airways obstruction is shown in Fig. 3.6.

THE FLOW–VOLUME LOOP

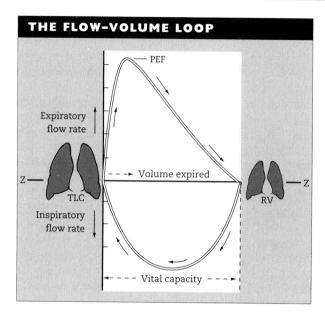

Fig. 3.5 The flow–volume loop. Air flow is represented on the vertical axis and lung volume on the horizontal axis. The line Z–Z represents zero flow. Expiratory flow appears above the line; inspiratory flow below. PEF, peak expiratory flow; TLC, total lung capacity; RV, residual volume.

entirely due to a lower concentration in the alveolar fraction which can be calculated, and the transfer of carbon monoxide can be derived.

Although $T_L$co and Kco are influenced by many factors (e.g. ventilation/perfusion (V/Q) imbalance, area of alveolar membrane, haemoglobin level) they are very useful measurements in clinical practice. A reduced $T_L$co is a strong indicator of a **parenchymal lung disorder** involving the alveoli or their blood supply. It is reduced, for example, in emphysema, fibrotic lung disease (e.g. cryptogenic fibrosing alveolitis) and pulmonary embolism. It may be increased in asthma (probably because of improved distribution of ventilation and perfusion), polycythaemia and alveolar haemorrhage (because extravasated blood binds carbon monoxide). Adjusting the $T_L$co for alveolar volume, giving the transfer coefficient (Kco), is useful in assessing if the reduced transfer factor is due to a loss of surface area for diffusion. For example, a patient who has had one lung removed will have a reduced $T_L$co but a normal Kco if the remaining lung is normal.

Respiratory muscle function tests

Weakness of the respiratory muscles causes a **restrictive ventilatory defect** with reduced total lung capacity and VC. Comparison of the VC in the erect and supine position is useful since the pressure of the abdominal contents on a weak diaphragm typically causes a fall of >30% in the **supine VC**. **Chest X-ray** often shows small lung fields with basal atelectasis and high hemidiaphragms. **Fluorosocopy screening** may show paradoxical upward movement of a weakened diaphragm during inspiration. When there is severe respiratory muscle weakness ventilatory failure develops with **hypercapnia**. Global respiratory muscle function may be assessed by measuring **mouth pressures**. Maximum inspiratory mouth pressure, P_I **max**, is measured during maximum inspiratory effort from residual volume against an obstructed airway using a mouthpiece and transducer device, and maximum expiratory mouth pressure, P_E **max**, is measured during a maximal expiratory effort from total lung capacity. The maximum **transdiaphragmatic**

CENTRAL AIRWAYS OBSTRUCTION

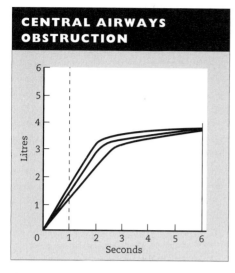

Fig. 3.6 Large (central) airways obstruction. Typical tracing obtained with a Vitalograph spirometer. The subject has made three maximal forced expirations. Each shows a striking straight section which then changes relatively abruptly, at about the same volume to follow the expected curve of the forced expiratory spirogram. The straight section is not as reproducible as a normal spirogram. A 'family' of similar tracings is thus obtained, each with straight and curved sections. *Explanation:* Over the straight section flow is limited by the fixed intrathoracic localized obstruction. This is little influenced by lung recoil so the critical flow is similar during expiration and the spirogram appears straight. A lung volume is eventually reached where maximum flow is even lower than that permitted by the central obstruction. The ordinary forced expiratory spirogram is described after this point. In the example shown there must be an element of diffuse airways obstruction, as forced expiratory time is somewhat prolonged (see Fig. 3.4c).

pressure generated during contraction can be measured in specialist laboratories using balloon catheters in the oesophagus and stomach.

Arterial blood gases

A **sample of arterial blood** may be obtained from any artery but the **radial artery** at the wrist or the **brachial artery** in the antecubital fossa are the sites most commonly used. Arterial puncture may be a painful procedure if there is difficulty in entering the artery quickly and directly so that **local anaesthetic** (e.g. 1% lignocaine) may be helpful. The blood enters the **heparinized needle** and syringe under its own pressure with a pulsatile action. The syringe containing the arterial blood is capped, placed in **ice** and analysed in the laboratory within 30 minutes of sampling.

The normal range for Po_2 in healthy young adults is about 11–14 kPa (83–105 mmHg), and for Pco_2 about 4.5–6 kPa (34–45 mmHg). Pco_2 is an index of alveolar ventilation and rises if there is a decrease in ventilation. Po_2 falls reciprocally with the increase in Pco_2 when there is alveolar underventilation but it also falls when there is V/Q mismatch, which is a common disturbance in lung disease.

Respiratory failure

Respiratory failure is a clinical term used to describe failure to maintain oxygenation (usually taken as an arbitrary cut-off point of Po_2 8.0 kPa (60 mmHg).
• *Type I respiratory failure* is hypoxaemia in the absence of hypercapnia and usually indicates a severe disturbance of V/Q relationships in the lungs. This pattern is seen in many conditions including pulmonary oedema, asthma, pulmonary embolism and lung fibrosis (Table 3.1).
• *Type II respiratory failure* is hypoxaemia with hypercapnia and indicates alveolar hypoventilation. This may occur from lack of neuromuscular control of ventilation (e.g. sedative overdose, cerebrovascular disease, myopathy) or from lung disease (e.g. COPD).

Oximetry

Oxygen saturation can be measured noninvasively and continuously using a pulse oximeter. Oxygenated blood appears red

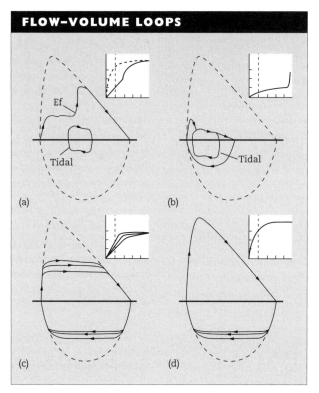

FLOW-VOLUME LOOPS

(a)

(b)

(c)

(d)

Fig. 3.7 Further flow–volume loops. The dotted outline represents a typical normal loop. The small graphs show the appearances of a forced expiration on a Vitalograph spirometer (as in Fig. 3.4).

(a) *Demonstration of maximum flow.* A normal individual makes an unhurried expiration from full inspiration and then about halfway through the vital capacity, a maximal expiratory effort (Ef) is made. The flow–volume tracing rejoins the maximum flow–volume curve which describes the highest flow which can be achieved at that lung volume. Also shown in (a) is the flow–volume loop of typical tidal breathing. At the resting lung volume there is an abundant reserve of both inspiratory and expiratory flow available.

(b) *Very severe airways obstruction* in an individual with emphysema. Maximum expiratory flow is very severely reduced. There is a brief peak (probably caused by airway collapse) after which flow falls very slowly. Also shown in (b) is a loop representing quiet tidal breathing. It is clear that every expiration is limited by maximum flow. Expiratory wheezing or purse lip breathing would be expected. There is some inspiratory reserve of flow but hardly any expiratory reserve. Ventilation could be increased slightly by adopting an even higher lung volume and by speeding up inspiration.

(c) *Fixed intrathoracic large airways obstruction:* for example, tracheal compression by a mediastinal tumour. Here the peak inspiratory and expiratory flows have been truncated in a characteristic pattern.

(d) *Variable extrathoracic obstruction.* Severe extrathoracic obstruction results in inspiratory collapse of the airway below the obstruction (but still outside the thorax). In this example expiration is normal, and this suggests a variable check-valve mechanism such as might be caused by bilateral vocal cord paralysis.

ARTERIAL GAS MEASUREMENTS

Po_2 kPa (mmHg)	Pco_2 kPa (mmHg)	A–a gradient kPa (mmHg)	Diagnosis
13 (98)	5 (38)	2 (15)	Normal
8 (60)	10 (75)	2 (15)	Sedative overdose Reduced ventilation Type 2 respiratory failure
6 (45)	4 (30)	10 (75)	Fibrotic lung disease V/Q mismatch Type 1 respiratory failure
15 (112)	3 (23)	2 (15)	Psychogenic hyperventilation
18 (135)	5 (38)	?	Patient not breathing air as $Po_2 + Pco_2 > 20$ kPa

A–a gradient: the alveolar to arterial gradient $= P_iO_2 - (Po_2 + Pco_2)$ (see Chapter 1).

Table 3.1 Examples of arterial gas measurements in various conditions.

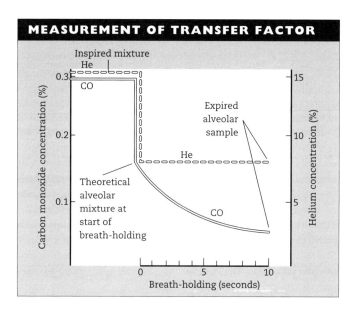

Fig. 3.8 Measurement of transfer factor by the single-breath method. Schematic representation of the helium and carbon monoxide concentrations in the inspired mixture and in alveolar air during breath-holding.

whereas reduced blood appears blue (clinical sign of cyanosis). An oximeter measures the ratio of oxygenated to total haemoglobin in arterial blood using a probe placed on a finger or ear lobe, which comprises two light-emitting diodes—one red and one infrared—and a detector. The light absorbed varies with each pulse, and measurement of light absorption at two points of the pulse wave allows the oxygen saturation of arterial blood to be determined. The accuracy of measurement is reduced if there is reduced arterial pulsation (e.g. low-output cardiac states) or increased venous pulsation (e.g. tricuspid regurgitation, venous congestion). Skin pigmentation or use of nail varnish may interfere with light transmission. Oximetry is also inaccurate in the presence of carboxyhaemoglobin (e.g. in carbon monoxide poisoning) which the oximeter detects as oxyhaemoglobin. The relationship of Po_2 to oxygen saturation is described by the **oxyhaemoglobin dissociation curve** (see Fig. 1.5). This curve is sigma-shaped so that oxygen saturation is closely related to Po_2 only over a short range of about 3–7 kPa. Above this level the dissociation curve begins to plateau and there is only a small increase in oxygen saturation as the Po_2 rises. Oximetry can reduce the need for arterial puncture, but arterial blood gas analysis is necessary to determine accurately the Po_2 on the plateau part of the oxyhaemoglobin dissociation curve, to measure carbon dioxide level and to assess acid–base status.

Acid–base balance

The three variables principally involved in acid–base balance in the body are **hydrogen ion concentration ([H+])**, Pco_2 and **bicarbonate [HCO$_3^-$]**. [H+] is generally expressed as pH which is the negative logarithm of [H+]. These variables are directly related to each other in terms of the Henderson–Hasselbalch equation $[H^+] \propto Pco_2/[HCO_3^-]$. There is a direct linear relationship between Pco_2 and [H+]. Bicarbonate concentration can be calcu-

lated if Pco_2 and pH are known or it can be measured directly: the **actual bicarbonate concentration**. **Standard bicarbonate** is a calculated value indicating what the bicarbonate would be at a standard Pco_2 of 5.3 kPa (40 mmHg). The **base excess** is a further parameter of the buffering capacity of the blood which recognizes the fact that there are other buffers apart from bicarbonate in the blood. Changes in pH which are caused primarily by an alteration in Pco_2 are termed **respiratory**, and are determined by **alveolar ventilation**. Changes in pH which are brought about by changes in bicarbonate concentration are termed **metabolic**. The renal tubules modulate bicarbonate concentration in response to the prevailing Pco_2 but this is a slow process.

• *Respiratory acidosis (acute)*: **pH reduced, Pco_2 raised, bicarbonate normal.** A reduction in alveolar ventilation causes an increase in arterial Pco_2. The pH falls in relation to the Pco_2. In the short term there is insufficient time for renal compensation by reabsorption of bicarbonate so that the bicarbonate concentration remains almost unchanged. This pattern is seen where there is acute hypoventilation, e.g. obstruction of the airway, overdose of sedative drugs or acute neurological damage.

• *Respiratory alkalosis*: **pH raised, Pco_2 reduced, bicarbonate normal.** Alveolar hyperventilation causes a fall in Pco_2 and a corresponding rise in pH. Bicarbonate concentration is virtually unchanged unless there is a longstanding respiratory alkalosis which is unusual. This pattern is seen in any form of acute hyperventilation, e.g. anxiety-related hyperventilation, salicylate poisoning, acute asthma.

• *Metabolic acidosis*: **pH reduced, Pco_2 reduced, bicarbonate reduced.** The primary disturbance is generally an increase in acid. This has an effect on the equilibrium $H^+ + HCO_3^- \rightleftharpoons H_2O + CO_2$ pushing it to the right. The carbon dioxide produced is removed by increased ventilation and the net result is a lowering of plasma bicarbonate. In practice the fall in pH causes respiratory stimulation so that carbon dioxide is promptly blown off. This respiratory compensation is an inevitable accompaniment of metabolic acidosis — acute and chronic — unless there is some other factor limiting ventilatory function or responsiveness. This pattern is seen in diabetic ketoacidosis, renal tubular acidosis, and acute circulatory failure and other forms of lactic acidosis.

• *Metabolic alkalosis*: **pH raised, $P\text{co}_2$ normal or slightly raised, bicarbonate raised.** An increase in bicarbonate concentration causes a rise in pH. The compensatory fall in alveolar ventilation is usually slight, therefore $P\text{co}_2$ usually increases a little. This pattern is seen where there has been administration of excessive alkali, loss of acid through vomiting, or reabsorption of bicarbonate (e.g. in hypokalaemia).

• *Chronic respiratory acidosis*: **pH normal or slightly reduced, $P\text{co}_2$ raised, bicarbonate raised.** If alveolar hypoventilation is sustained for some days, renal tubular reabsorption of bicarbonate will achieve significant elevation of plasma bicarbonate level tending to correct the acidosis (chronic compensated respiratory acidosis). This pattern is seen in any cause of sustained hypoventilation, e.g. COPD, chronic neuromuscular disease.

• *Mixed disturbances*: **mixed respiratory and metabolic disturbances** are common and there are usually a number of possible explanations, therefore it is essential to consider all the clinical details before interpreting the acid–base data. Figure 3.9 shows the situations that may arise in complex acid–base disturbances. For example, point (a) in Fig. 3.9 (low pH, normal $P\text{co}_2$, low bicarbonate) indicates a mixed metabolic and respiratory acidosis. This could arise in a patient with acute pulmonary oedema who is hypoxaemic with low cardiac output. The metabolic acidosis results from lactic acidosis and the patient's ability to hyperventilate is compromised. The same situation could arise in a totally different set of clinical circumstances (e.g. a patient in renal failure given a narcotic sedative suppressing ventilatory response to acidosis) so that acid–base

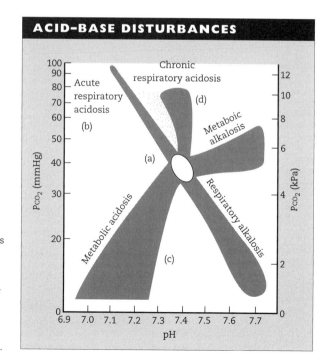

ACID-BASE DISTURBANCES

Fig. 3.9 Acid–base disturbances. The oval indicates the normal position. The shaded areas indicate the direction of observed 'pure' or uncomplicated disturbances of acid–base balance. Bicarbonate levels are omitted for clarity. Letters (a)–(d) are referred to in the text (see *Mixed disturbances*).

data have limited diagnostic potential considered alone. Point (b) could represent the situation soon after a cardiac arrest where severe lactic acidosis exists and ventilation has been insufficient. Point (c) could represent the situation in severe aspirin poisoning where aspirin-induced hyperventilation has been complicated by aspirin-induced metabolic acidosis. Point (d) could represent the situation in an individual with chronic hypercapnia due to COPD who is stimulated to increase ventilation by a pulmonary embolism.

Further reading

Cotes JE. Lung Function: Assessment and Application in Medicine. Oxford: Blackwell Scientific Publications, 1993.

Flenley DC. Interpretation of blood-gas and acid–base data. Br J Hosp Med 1978; 20: 384–94.

Gibson GJ. Clinical Tests of Respiratory Function. Oxford: Chapman and Hall, 1996.

Gibson GJ. Measurement of respiratory muscle strength. Respir Med 1995; 89: 529–35.

Hanning CD, Alexander-Williams JM. Pulse oximetry: a practical review. BMJ 1995; 311: 367–70.

CHAPTER 4

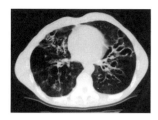

Radiology of the Chest

Chest X-ray

The chest X-ray plays a key role in the investigation of respiratory disease. The standard view is the erect, **postero-anterior (PA) chest X-ray** taken at full inspiration with the X-ray beam passing from back to front. A **lateral X-ray** gives a better view of lesions lying behind the heart or diaphragm, which may not be visible on a PA X-ray, and allows abnormalities to be viewed in a further dimension. Supine and **anteroposterior (AP) views** are usually taken at the bedside using mobile equipment in patients who are too ill to be brought to the X-ray department. AP films are less satisfactory in defining many abnormalities, producing magnification of the cardiac outline, for example.

The main landmarks of the normal chest X-ray are shown in Figs 4.1 and 4.2. X-rays should be examined both close up and from a short distance on a viewing box in an area with reduced background lighting. It is important to confirm the name and date on the X-ray and to check the technical quality of the film. Symmetry between the medial end of both clavicles and the thoracic spine confirms that the film has been taken without any rotation artefact. If the film has been taken in full inspiration the right hemidiaphragm is normally intersected by the anterior part of the sixth rib. The vertebral bodies are usually visible through the cardiac shadow if the X-ray exposure is satisfactory. It is helpful to examine the film systematically to avoid missing useful information. The shape and bony structures of the chest wall should be surveyed and the position of the hemidiaphragms and trachea noted. The heart's shape and size and the appearances of the mediastinum and hilar shadows are examined. The size, shape and disposition of the vascular shadows are noted and the pattern of the lung markings in different zones carefully compared. Any abnormality detected should be analysed in detail and interpreted in the context of all clinical information. It is often helpful to obtain previous X-rays or to monitor the evolution of abnormalities over time on follow-up X-rays. Some of the radiological features of the major lung diseases are shown in individual chapters. In some circumstances chest X-ray abnormalities follow a specific pattern which allows a differential diagnosis to be outlined.

Abnormal features

Collapse

Obstruction of a bronchus by a carcinoma, foreign body (e.g. inhaled peanut) or mucus plug causes loss of aeration with '**loss of volume**' and collapse of the lung distal to the obstruction. Collapse of each individual lobe of the lung produces its own particular appearance on chest X-ray (Figs 4.3 and 4.4) with **shift of landmarks** such as the mediastinum resulting from loss of volume. Obstruction of a main bronchus usually causes obvious asymme-

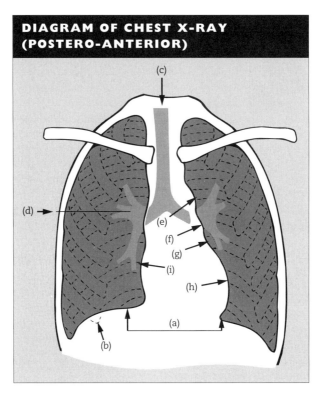

DIAGRAM OF CHEST X-RAY (POSTERO-ANTERIOR)

Fig. 4.1 Diagram of chest X-ray (PA view). The right hemidiaphragm is 1–3 cm higher than the left (a) and on full inspiration it is intersected by the shadow of the anterior part of the sixth rib (b). The trachea (c) is vertical and central or very slightly to the right. The horizontal fissure (d) is found in the position shown, or slightly lower and should be truly horizontal. It is a very valuable marker of change in volume of any part of the right lung. The left border of the cardiac shadow comprises: (e) aorta; (f) pulmonary artery; (g) concavity overlying the left atrial appendage; (h) left ventricle. The right border of the cardiac shadow normally overlies the right atrium (i) and above that the superior vena cava.

try (Fig. 4.5). **Compensatory expansion** of other lobes may result in increased transradiency of adjacent areas of the lung. In right middle lobe collapse there may be little to see on a PA X-ray apart from lack of definition of the right heart border. This is a useful sign which helps to distinguish it from lower lobe collapse where the right border of the heart remains clearly defined. Left lower lobe collapse is manifest as a triangular area of increased density behind the heart shadow, often with a shift of the heart shadow to the left and increased transradiency of the left hemithorax due to compensatory expansion of the left upper lobe. Collapse is a sinister sign often indicating an obstructing carcinoma which may be confirmed by bronchoscopy.

Consolidation

Air in the lungs appears black on X-ray. Consolidation appears as **areas of opacification** sometimes conforming to the outline of a lobe or segment of lung in which the air has been replaced by an inflammatory exudate (e.g. pneumonia), fluid (e.g. pulmonary oedema), blood (e.g. pulmonary haemorrhage) or tumour (e.g. alveolar cell carcinoma). Bronchi containing air passing through the consolidated

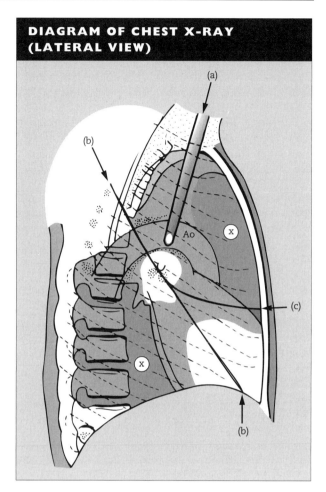

Fig. 4.2 Diagram of chest X-ray (lateral view). (a) Trachea. (b) Oblique fissure. (c) Horizontal fissure. It is useful to note that in a normal lateral view the radiodensity of the lung field above and in front of the cardiac shadow is about the same as that below and behind (x). Ao, aorta.

lung are sometimes clearly visible as black tubes of air against the white background of the consolidated lung: **air bronchograms** (see Fig. 18.2, p. 180). Structures such as the heart, mediastinum and diaphragm are usually clearly outlined as a silhouette on an X-ray because of the contrast between the blackness of aerated lung and the whiteness of these structures. When there is abnormal shadowing in the lung adjacent to these structures there is loss of the sharp outline, and this is often referred to as the **silhouette sign** (Fig. 4.6).

Pulmonary masses (Table 4.1)

Various descriptive terms such as 'rounded opacity', 'nodule' or 'coin lesion' are used to refer to pulmonary masses. Carcinoma of the lung is the most important cause of a mass on chest X-ray but several other diseases may cause a similar appearance. Features such as **cavitation, calcification, rate of growth**, the presence of **associated abnormalities** (e.g. lymph node enlargement) and whether the lesion is **solitary** or whether **multiple** lesions are present, may provide clues to diagnosis. However, these features are often not reliable indicators of aetiology, and the X-ray appearances must be interpreted in the context of all the clinical information. Further investigations such as computed tomography

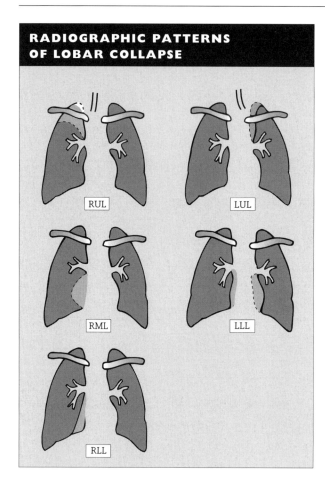

RADIOGRAPHIC PATTERNS OF LOBAR COLLAPSE

RUL   LUL

RML   LLL

RLL

Fig. 4.3 Radiographic patterns of lobar collapse. Collapsed lobes occupy a surprisingly small volume and are commonly overlooked on the chest X-ray. Note the position of the diaphragms in each case. Helpful information may be provided by the position of the trachea, the hilar vascular shadows and the horizontal fissure. RUL, right upper lobe; RML, right middle lobe; RLL, right lower lobe; LUL, left upper lobe; LLL, left lower lobe.

PULMONARY MASSES

Neoplastic
Primary bronchial carcinoma
Metastatic carcinoma
Benign tumours (hamartoma)

Non-neoplastic
Tuberculoma
Lung abscess
Hydatid cyst
Pulmonary infarct
Arteriovenous malformation
Encysted interlobar effusion
    ('pseudotumour')
Rheumatoid nodule

Table 4.1 Causes of pulmonary masses.

(CT) and biopsy (bronchoscopic, percutaneous, surgical) are often necessary.

Cavitation

Cavitation is the presence of an area of radiolucency within a mass lesion. It is a feature of **bronchial carcinoma** (particularly squamous carcinoma) (Fig. 4.7), **tuberculosis, lung abscess, pulmonary infarcts, Wegener's granulomatosis** (see p. 165) and some **pneumonias** (e.g. *Staphylococcus aureus*, *Klebsiella pneumoniae*).

Fibrosis

Localized fibrosis produces **streaky shadows** with evidence of **traction** upon neighbouring structures. Upper lobe fibrosis causes traction

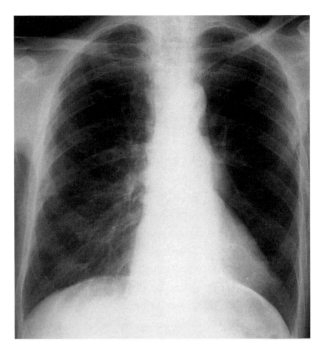

Fig. 4.4 Left lower lobe collapse. The left lower lobe has collapsed medially and posteriorly and appears as a dense white triangular area behind the heart close to the mediastinum. The remainder of the left lung appears hyperlucent due to compensatory expansion. Bronchoscopy showed an adenocarcinoma occluding the left lower lobe bronchus.

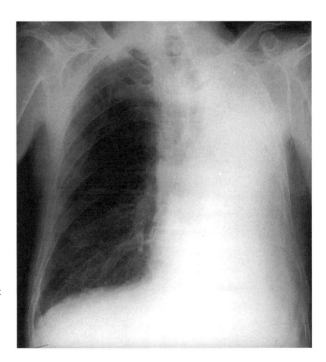

Fig. 4.5 Left lung collapse. There is complete opacification of the left hemithorax with shift of the mediastinum to the left. Bronchoscopy showed a small-cell carcinoma occluding the left main bronchus.

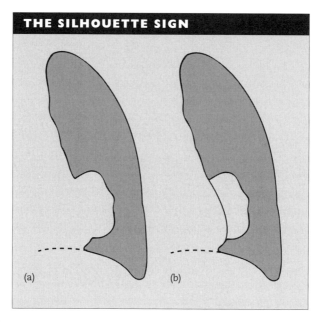

THE SILHOUETTE SIGN

(a)   (b)

Fig. 4.6 The silhouette sign. Diagram showing abnormal lung shadowing in the left lower zone, where the sharp outline of mediastinal structures or diaphragm is lost because of abnormal lung opacification. It can be concluded that the shadowing is immediately adjacent to the structure (and vice versa). In example (a) the shadowing must be anterior and next to the heart, as the sharp outline of the heart is lost. In (b) it must be posterior as the heart outline is preserved.

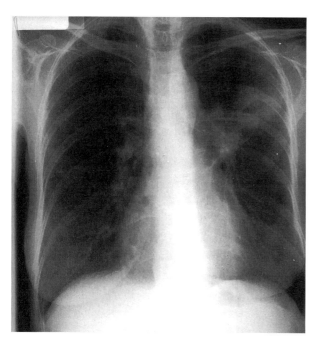

Fig. 4.7 A cavitating lesion in the left upper lobe. A cavity appears as an area of radiolucency (black) within an opacity (white). Sputum cytology showed cells from a squamous carcinoma. Computed tomography showed left hilar and subcarinal lymphadenopathy.

upon the trachea and elevation of the hilar vascular shadows. Generalized interstitial fibrosis produces a hazy shadowing with a **fine reticular (net-like)** or **nodular pattern** (see Chapter 14). Advanced interstitial fibrosis results in a honeycomb pattern with diffuse opacification containing multiple circular translucencies a few millimetres in diameter.

Mediastinal masses

Metastatic tumour or lymphomatous involvement of the mediastinal lymph nodes are the commonest causes of mediastinal masses but there are a number of other diseases which may cause mediastinal masses (Fig. 4.8). Thymic tumours, thyroid masses and dermoid cysts are most commonly situated in the anterior mediastinum whereas neural lesions (e.g. neurofibroma), and oesophageal cysts are often situated posteriorly. Aneurysmal enlargement of the aorta or ventricle may produce masses in the middle compartment of the mediastinum. CT scans are helpful in delineating the anatomy of mediastinal lesions. Thoracotomy with surgical excision is often necessary.

Ultrasonography of the chest

Normal air-filled lung does not transmit high-frequency sound waves so that ultrasonography is not useful in assessing disease of lung parenchyma. It may be helpful in assessing lesions of the pleura and is particularly useful for localizing loculated pleural effusions.

Computed tomography

CT scanning uses a technique of multiple projection with reconstruction of the image from

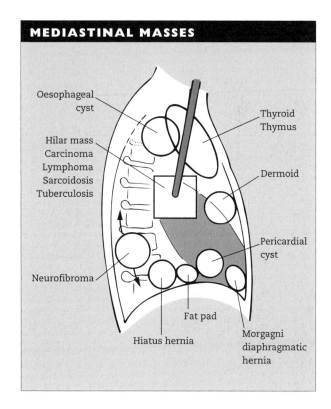

MEDIASTINAL MASSES

Oesophageal cyst

Hilar mass
Carcinoma
Lymphoma
Sarcoidosis
Tuberculosis

Thyroid
Thymus

Dermoid

Pericardial cyst

Neurofibroma

Fat pad

Hiatus hernia

Morgagni diaphragmatic hernia

Fig. 4.8 Mediastinal masses. Diagram of lateral view of the chest, indicating the sites favoured by some of the commoner mediastinal masses.

MEDIASTINAL STRUCTURES

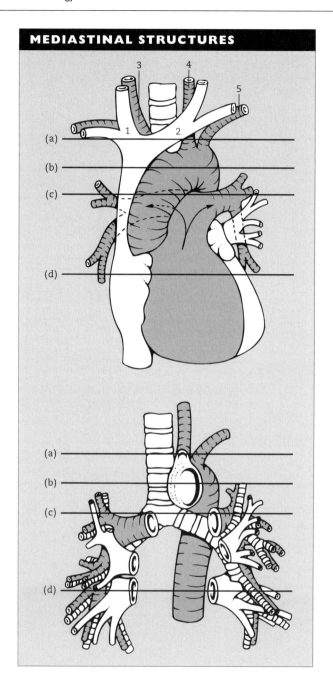

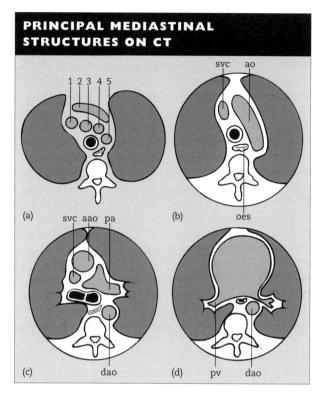

PRINCIPAL MEDIASTINAL STRUCTURES ON CT

Fig. 4.10 Principal mediastinal structures on computed tomography (CT). The sections (a) to (d) are at levels (a) to (d) in Fig. 4.9. The sections should be regarded as being viewed from below **(i.e. the left of the thorax is on the right of the figure).** (a) *Section above the aortic arch.* Many large vessels and an anterior sausage shape are seen; the trachea has not bifurcated (black circle). Numerals refer to Fig. 4.9 and its legend. (b) *Section at the level of aortic arch.* A large oblique sausage shape representing the aortic arch is seen (ao); svc, superior vena cava; oes, oesophagus which is visible in all of the sections. (c) *Section below the aortic arch.* Both ascending (aao) and descending (dao) aortas are visible, the trachea is bifurcating and the pulmonary arteries are seen; pa, left pulmonary artery. (d) *Section at the level of pulmonary veins (pv).* Lower lobe intrapulmonary arteries and bronchi are not shown in the diagram.

Fig. 4.9 Mediastinal structures. Principal blood vessels and airways.
Above: Heart and major blood vessels showing the aorta curling over the bifurcation of the pulmonary trunk into left and right pulmonary arteries (arrows). The horizontal lines (a) to (d) indicate the levels of the computed tomography (CT) sections illustrated in Fig. 4.10. 1, right brachiocephalic vein; 2, left brachiocephalic vein; 3, innominate or brachiocephalic artery; 4, left common carotid artery; 5, left subclavian artery. *Below:* Structures with the heart removed. The aorta curls over the left main bronchus which lies behind the left pulmonary artery. Pulmonary arteries are shown shaded, pulmonary veins unshaded and bronchi are shown striped. In general the arteries loop downwards, like a handlebar moustache; veins radiate towards a lower common destination—the left atrium. The veins are applied to the front of the arteries and bronchi and take a slightly different path to the respective lung segments. On the right, the order of structures from front to back is vein–artery–bronchus; on the left the pulmonary artery loops over the left upper lobe bronchus and descends behind so that the order is vein–bronchus–artery.

X-ray detectors by a computer so that structures can be displayed in cross-section. A number of different techniques can be used depending on the area of interest, and interpretation of CT images will normally be carried out by an expert radiologist. CT scanning is particularly useful in providing a detailed cross-sectional image of mediastinal disease which is often difficult to assess on plain chest X-ray. Figure 4.9 shows the principal mediastinal structures with horizontal lines indicating the levels of the CT sections illustrated diagrammatically in Fig. 4.10. CT scanning is particularly important in the staging of the lung cancer (see Chapter 13), and has virtually replaced bronchography (instillation of radiocontrast dye into the bronchial tree) in detecting and determining the extent of bronchiectasis (see Chapter 9). High-resolution CT scans are much more sensitive than plain X-ray in assessing the lung parenchyma and can provide a detailed image of emphysema (see Chapter 12) and interstitial lung disease. A 'ground glass' appearance on a high-resolution CT scan of a patient with cryptogenic fibrosing alveolitis, for example, corresponds to a cellular pattern on histology whereas a 'reticular pattern' often indicates fibrosis with less active inflammation and less response to steroids (see Chapter 14). Some modern CT scanners have the capacity to perform very rapid spiral images and this imaging technique combined with injection of radiocontrast material into a peripheral vein can be used to identify emboli in central pulmonary arteries in thromboembolic disease (see Chapter 16).

Further reading

Hansell DM. Thoracic imaging. In: Brewis RAL, Corrin B, Geddes DM, Gibson GJ, eds. *Respiratory Medicine*. London: WB Saunders Co., 1995: 278–317.

Modini C, Passariello R, Iascone C et al. TNM staging in lung cancer: role of computed tomography. *J. Thorac Cardiovasc Surg* 1982; **48**: 569–73.

Patel PR. *Lecture Notes on Radiology*. Oxford: Blackwell Science, 1998: 19–60.

Remy-Jardin M, Remy J, Wattinne L et al. Central pulmonary thromboembolism: diagnosis with spiral volumatic CT with the single-breath-hold technique—comparison with pulmonary angiography. *Radiology* 1992; **185**: 381–7.

Wells AV, Hansell, DM, Rubens MB. The predictive value of high resolution computed tomography in fibrosing alveolitis. *Am Rev Respir Dis* 1993; **148**: 1076–80.

CHAPTER 5

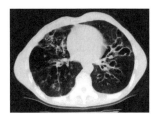

Upper Respiratory Tract Infections

Introduction

Acute upper respiratory tract infections (URTI) are a very common cause of morbidity, visits to doctors, and absence from school or work. They are the commonest respiratory complaint accounting for about **9% of all consultations in general practice**. A child suffers about eight, and an adult about four respiratory infections each year. Although unpleasant, most URTIs are mild and self-limiting, but a small number give rise to serious problems, most notably acute epiglottitis in children and influenza A in elderly patients debilitated by chronic underlying disease. Difficulties arise in distinguishing URTIs from more serious lower respiratory tract infections such as pneumonia (Fig. 5.1), and alertness combined with careful assessment and clinical judgement are required. Most URTIs are of viral origin but a variety of viruses and bacteria may produce the same clinical pattern of illness (e.g. pharyngitis, sinusitis).

Common cold

The common cold (coryza) is an acute illness characterized by rhinorrhoea, sneezing, nasal obstruction and sore throat (pharyngitis) with minimal fever or systemic symptoms. It may be caused by a number of different viruses including **rhinoviruses, coronaviruses, res-**piratory **syncytial, parainfluenza** and **influenza viruses**. Infection is transmitted by droplet spread, and attack rates are highest in young children attending school who then transmit infection to their parents and siblings at home. The multiplicity of viral strains prevents the development of immunity. The bacterial flora of the nasopharynx remains unchanged for the first few days of the illness but then may show an increase in the number of *Haemophilus influenzae* and *Streptococcus pneumoniae* organisms, and there is the potential for secondary bacterial infection to occur with extension of infection beyond the nasopharynx giving rise to sinusitis, otitis media, bronchitis or pneumonia. No specific treatment is possible for the common cold but symptoms are often alleviated by use of paracetamol or aspirin.

Pharyngitis

Pharyngitis may occur as part of the common cold or as a separate illness. Most cases are due to **viruses** (Table 5.1) but pharyngitis may also be caused by group A β-**haemolytic streptococci, *Mycoplasma pneumoniae*** or ***Chlamydia pneumoniae***, for example. The patient complains of a sore throat and there is erythema of the pharynx often with enlargement of the tonsils. **Infectious mononucleosis** ('glandular fever') often involves pharyngitis

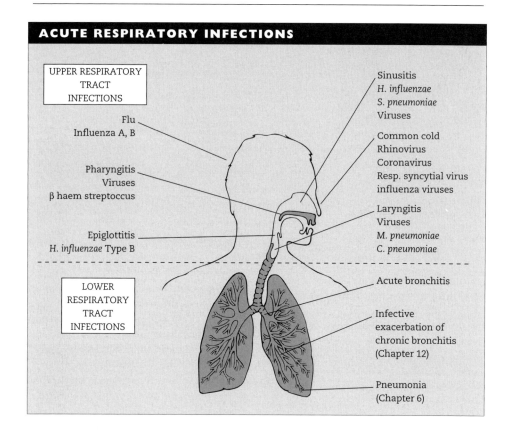

ACUTE RESPIRATORY INFECTIONS

UPPER RESPIRATORY
TRACT
INFECTIONS

Flu
Influenza A, B

Pharyngitis
Viruses
β haem streptoccus

Epiglottitis
H. influenzae Type B

LOWER
RESPIRATORY
TRACT
INFECTIONS

Sinusitis
H. influenzae
S. pneumoniae
Viruses

Common cold
Rhinovirus
Coronavirus
Resp. syncytial virus
influenza viruses

Laryngitis
Viruses
M. pneumoniae
C. pneumoniae

Acute bronchitis

Infective
exacerbation of
chronic bronchitis
(Chapter 12)

Pneumonia
(Chapter 6)

Fig. 5.1 Acute respiratory infections.

but is also associated with lymphadenopathy and splenomegaly. Most cases are caused by the Epstein–Barr virus. A blood film may show atypical mononuclear cells and the Monospot or heterophile antibody tests are positive. Characteristically, patients with infectious mononucleosis develop a rash if given amoxycillin as treatment of pharyngitis. It is not possible to distinguish between viral and bacterial pharyngitis on clinical grounds. β-haemolytic streptococci may be found on microbiology of a throat swab but this does not differentiate between active infection and a carriage state. Even when pharyngitis is due to bacterial infection antibiotics are not usually necessary as the illness tends to be self-limiting. Local extension of infection may result in otitis media, tonsillitis

or quinsy (peritonsillar abscess). Streptococcal infection may be complicated by glomerulonephritis or rheumatic fever but these are rare nowadays. Antibiotic treatment of pharyngitis is usually only given to severe or complicated cases. Streptococci are sensitive to penicillin V or amoxycillin. *Mycoplasma pneumoniae* or *Chlamydia pneumoniae* require a tetracycline or macrolide antibiotic (e.g. erythromycin, clarithromycin).

Sinusitis

Infection of the maxillary sinuses causes facial pain, nasal obstruction and discharge, often accompanied by fever and malaise. A variety of organisms may cause sinusitis including respiratory **viruses**, ***Haemophilus influenzae***, ***Streptococcus pneumoniae***, **Staphylococ-**

RESPIRATORY VIRUSES

Virus	Disease	Notes
Rhinovirus	Common cold, pharyngitis, chronic bronchitic exacerbations	More than 100 serotypes; identification and study difficult
Coronavirus	Common cold	Numerous serotypes; identification difficult
Adenovirus	Pharyngitis, conjunctivitis, severe bronchitis in childhood, rarely severe pneumonia	About 30 serotypes
Respiratory syncytial virus	Bronchiolitis in infants, common cold in adults	One serotype, winter epidemics
Influenza A	Influenza—may be severe	Epidemics, continuous antigenic variation
Influenza B	Influenza	Milder illness, minor epidemics
Parainfluenza	Croup, other upper respiratory tract infections, some bronchiolitis	Serotypes 1–4, a and b
Measles	Measles, severe illness with pneumonia in immunocompromised	Vaccination effective
Cytomegalovirus	Silent infection or minor respiratory illness, pneumonia in immunosuppressed	One serotype
Herpes simplex	Stomatitis, rarely pharyngitis, pneumonia in immunosuppressed	One serotype, severe infection treatable with acyclovir or vidarabine
Herpes zoster	Pneumonia in adult infection	Severe infection treatable with acyclovir, leaves scattered calcific lesions
Coxsackie, enteroviruses and ECHO viruses	Minor part in respiratory infection, Coxsackie A may cause herpangina; B causes 'pleurodynia' and pericarditis/myocarditis	Local epidemics
Epstein–Barr (EB) virus	Pharyngitis, lymphadenitis, infectious mononucleosis	Heterophile antibody test, typical blood picture

Table 5.1 Principal respiratory viruses.

cus aureus, and **anaerobic bacteria**. In chronic sinusitis X-rays may show mucosal thickening, opacification, or the presence of a fluid level in the sinus. Recurrent sinusitis may be accompanied by more widespread respiratory tract infection in patients with bronchiectasis due to cystic fibrosis, hypogammaglobulinaemia or ciliary dyskinesia. Post-nasal drip from sinusitis is irritating to the larynx and is quite a common cause of a persistent cough. Sinusitis is usually treated with antibiotics (e.g. amoxycillin, trimethoprim), nasal decongestants (e.g. ephedrine) and analgesia (e.g. paracetamol). Surgical drainage may be necessary for relief of chronic sinusitis.

Acute laryngitis

This term is used when temporary hoarseness or loss of voice occurs with pharyngitis or the common cold, and is due to oedema of the vocal cords. No treatment is necessary.

Croup

Croup (acute laryngotracheobronchitis) is usually caused by **viruses** such as parainfluenza virus, respiratory syncytial virus, influenza A and B, rhinoviruses, adenovirus and measles. Characteristically the child develops a harsh barking cough with an upper respiratory infection and this may progress to stridor. Often no treatment is required but some children develop more severe lower respiratory infections and progressive respiratory distress requiring intubation and ventilation. Oral prednisolone is sometimes beneficial in severe croup and nebulized high-dose budesonide may be associated with more rapid recovery in less severely affected patients.

Acute epiglottitis

Epiglottitis is a very serious disease which is usually caused by virulent strains of *Haemophilus influenzae* **type b**, and there is often an accompanying septicaemia. Death may result from occlusion of the airway by the inflamed oedematous epiglottis. It is commonest in children of about 2–3 years of age, but cases have also occurred in adults. The patient is ill with pyrexia, sore throat, laryngitis and painful dysphagia. Symptoms of upper airway obstruction may develop rapidly with stridor and respiratory distress. A lateral neck X-ray may show the epiglottic swelling. Blood cultures often isolate *Haemophilus influenzae* type B. Patients with suspected epiglottitis should be admitted to hospital and attempts at examining the upper airway should only be performed when facilities are available for tracheal intubation and ventilation. Because of possible amoxycillin resistance chloramphenicol or cefuroxime are appropriate antibiotics.

Influenza

Influenza is an acute illness characterized by pyrexia, malaise, myalgia, headache and prostration as well as upper respiratory symptoms. Lethargy and depression may persist for several days afterwards. Although the term 'flu' is used very loosely by the public, it is the systemic features which characterize true infection with the influenza viruses. Influenza virus type A undergoes frequent spontaneous changes in its haemagglutinin and neuraminidase surface antigens. Minor changes, referred to as '**antigenic drift**', result in outbreaks of influenza in the winter months each year. Major changes, referred to as '**antigenic shift**', result in epidemics and pandemics of infection reflecting the lack of immunity in the population to the new strain. Type B is more antigenically stable and produces less severe disease. Type C causes only mild sporadic cases of upper respiratory infection.

Influenza is highly infectious so that all members of a household often become ill together. Outbreaks of influenza cause considerable morbidity even in healthy adults. It is usually a self-limiting illness but can be complicated by bronchitis, otitis media and secondary bacterial pneumonia (e.g. *Staphylococcus aureus*, *Streptococcus pneumoniae* or *Haemophilus influenzae*). The greatest morbidity and mortality occur in patients who are elderly with underlying cardiac or respiratory disease. Primary influenzal pneumonia is rare but severe.

The diagnosis of influenza can be confirmed by immunofluorescent microscopy of nasal secretions or by serology. Although anti-viral treatments with amantadine or ribavirin have been tried there is no effective specific treatment of influenza. Use of aspirin or paracetamol relieves symptoms. Antibiotics are used when there are features of secondary bacterial infection (e.g. otitis media, sinusitis). Pneumonia associated with influenza may be severe and requires treatment with broad-spectrum antibiotics including flucloxacillin because of the risk of *Staphylococcus aureus* infection.

Influenza vaccination

The influenza vaccine is prepared each year using the virus strains most likely to be prevalent that year. The vaccine contains inactivated virus and is about 70–80% effective in protecting against infection. Where infection occurs despite vaccination it is usually less severe and associated with less morbidity and mortality than the disease seen in unvaccinated patients. Selective immunization is recommended to protect those most at risk of serious illness or death from influenza. Annual vaccination is recommended for those with chronic respiratory disease (e.g. chronic obstructive pulmonary disease, asthma, bronchiectasis, etc.), chronic heart disease, renal failure, diabetes mellitus, immunosuppression, and for elderly patients living in nursing homes.

Adverse reactions to influenza vaccine are usually mild consisting of fever and malaise in some patients and local reactions at the site of injection. The vaccine is contra-indicated in patients with egg allergy. Patients should be advised that the vaccine will not protect them from all respiratory viruses.

Further reading

Husby S, Agertoft L, Mortensen S, Pedersen S. Treatment of croup with nebulised steroid (budesonide): a double-blind placebo controlled study. *Arch Dis Child* 1993; **68**: 352–6.

Little PS, Williamson I, Shvartzman P. Are antibiotics appropriate for sore throats? *BMJ* 1994; **309**: 1010–12.

Mansel JK, Rosenow EC, Smith TF, Martin JW. *Mycoplasma pneumoniae. Chest* 1989; **95**: 639–46.

Vernon DD, Sarnaik AP. Acute epiglottitis in children: a conservative approach to diagnosis and management. *Crit Care Med* 1986; **14**: 23–25.

Wilson R. Influenza vaccination. *Thorax* 1994; **49**: 1079–80.

CHAPTER 6

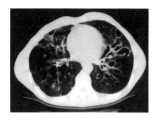

Pneumonia

Introduction

Pneumonia is a general term denoting inflammation of the gas exchange region of the lung. Usually it implies **parenchymal lung inflammation caused by infection**, and the term 'pneumonitis' is used to denote inflammation due to physical, chemical or allergic processes. Pneumonia is an important cause of morbidity and mortality in all age groups. Globally it is estimated that 5 million children under the age of 5 years die from pneumonia each year (95% in the developing countries). In the UK about 1 in 1000 of the population are admitted to hospital with pneumonia each year and the mortality in these patients is about 10%. There are about 3000 deaths from pneumonia each year in the age group 15–55 years. About 25% of all deaths in the elderly are related to pneumonia, although this is often the terminal illness in a patient with serious concomitant disease.

Classification in relation to clinical context (Fig. 6.1)

Pneumonia is the result of a complex interaction between the **patient**, the **environment** and the **infecting organism**. The clinical context, the patient's previous health status and the virulence of the organism are key elements determining the pattern of the disease.

The clinical approach to pneumonia therefore focuses on the circumstances of the illness:

- site of infection in the respiratory tract;
- age of the patient;
- community- or hospital-acquired infection;
- concurrent disease;
- environmental and geographical factors;
- severity of the illness;
- microbiology of the pneumonia.

Site of infection

The term 'chest infection' is an imprecise term often used by lay people to refer to nonspecific respiratory symptoms. In assessing and treating respiratory tract infections it is important to define the site of infection as clearly as possible. **Upper respiratory tract infections** (above the larynx) are often viral in origin and self-limiting, not requiring treatment (see Chapter 5). **Lower respiratory tract infections** may affect the bronchial tree as **bronchitis**, or the lung parenchyma as **pneumonia**. Infective exacerbations of chronic bronchitis (see Chapter 12) are often caused by organisms of low virulence (e.g. non-typeable *Haemophilus influenzae*) when the patient's defences against infection are compromised by smoking-induced damage to the bronchial mucosa. Penetration of antibiotics into the scarred mucosa and viscid secretions may be difficult. Extension of bronchial infection into the surrounding lung parenchyma is often referred to as **bronchopneumonia**.

LIKELY CAUSES OF PNEUMONIA

Previously well infant
1 RSV
2 Adenovirus and other viruses
3 Bacterial

Previously ill infant
1 *Staphylococcus*
2 E. coli and Gram-negative bacteria
3 Viruses and opportunistic organisms

Children
1 Viruses
2 *Pneumococcus*
3 *Mycoplasma*
4 Others

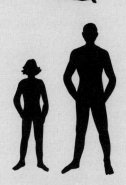

Previously fit adults
1 *Pneumococcus*
2 *Mycoplasma*
3 *H. influenzae*
4 Viruses
5 *Staphylococcus*
6 *Legionella*
7 Others

**Previous respiratory illness;
elderly and debilitated**
1 *Pneumococcus*
2 *H. influenzae*
3 *Staphylococcus*
4 *Klebsiella* and
   Gram-negative organisms

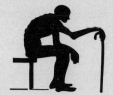

If no response think of:
TB, *Mycoplasma*, *Legionella*,
carcinoma

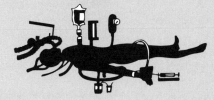

**Severely immunocompromised
and AIDS** (see Chapter 8):
1 Pneumocystis pneumonia
2 Cytomegalovirus
3 Adenovirus
4 Herpes simplex
5 Bacteria (*Legionella*,
   Staphylococcus, *Pneumococcus*)
6 Opportunistic mycobacteria;
   tuberculosis

Hospital-acquired pneumonia
1 Gram-negative bacteria
   (*Pseudomonas*, *Klebsiella*,
   Proteus)
2 *Staphylococcus*
3 *Pneumococcus*
4 Anaerobic bacteria, fungi
5 NB aspiration pneumonia
6 Others

Fig. 6.1 Likely causes of pneumonia in different clinical circumstances. Age and previous health are important factors.

Infection of the lung parenchyma with extensive consolidation of a lobe of a lung — **lobar pneumonia** — is usually caused by organisms of greater virulence (e.g. *Streptococcus pneumoniae*). Infection may spread to the pleura resulting in **empyema**, or to the blood stream causing **septicaemia**.

Age of the patient

In **children** under the age of 2 years pneumonia is more commonly due to viruses such as respiratory syncytial virus (RSV), adenovirus, influenza and parainfluenza viruses. *Chlamydia trachomatis* infection may be transmitted to the infant from the mother's genital tract during birth resulting in pneumonia. In older children and **adults** of all ages *Streptococcus pneumoniae* is the commonest cause of primary pneumonia. *Mycoplasma pneumoniae* infection is rare in the elderly and particularly affects young adults. The incidence of pneumonia increases greatly in the **elderly** and the high frequency of underlying chronic diseases (e.g. chronic obstructive pulmonary disease (COPD), heart failure) in this group is associated with a high mortality.

Community- or hospital-acquired pneumonia

The characteristics of the patients and the spectrum of pathogens differ greatly depending on whether pneumonia is contracted in the community or in hospital. When pneumonia is acquired in the community it may be a primary infection in a previously healthy individual or it may occur in association with concomitant disease (e.g. COPD), but a few pathogens (notably *Streptococcus pneumoniae*) account for the majority of cases and Gram-negative organisms are rare. Most patients are treated at home with only about 25% needing hospital admission. The most important organisms identified as causing **community-acquired pneumonia** are:

Streptococcus pneumoniae	60%
Mycoplasma pneumoniae	10%
Haemophilus influenzae	10%
Viruses (e.g. influenza)	10%

Staphylococcus aureus	3%
Legionella pneumophila	2%
Others (e.g. *Chlamydia pneumoniae*)	5%

Hospital-acquired (nosocomial pneumonia) is defined as pneumonia developing 2 or more days after admission to hospital for some other reason. It is therefore a secondary infection in patients with other illnesses. In these circumstances Gram-negative organisms (e.g. *Pseudomonas aeruginosa, Escherichia coli*) are the most important pathogens. A variety of factors, including use of broad-spectrum antibiotics and impaired host defences, promote the colonization of the nasopharynx of hospitalized patients with Gram-negative organisms. Aspiration of infected nasopharyngeal secretions into the lower respiratory tract is facilitated by factors which compromise the defence mechanisms of the lung, e.g. endotracheal intubation in intensive care, impaired cough associated with anaesthesia, surgery or cerebrovascular disease. The spectrum of causative organisms varies depending on the exact circumstances but the commonest pathogens in **hospital-acquired pneumonia** are:

Gram-negative bacteria	50%
Staphylococcus aureus	20%
Streptococcus pneumoniae	15%
Anaerobes and fungi	10%
Others	5%

Concurrent disease

Alcohol misuse, malnutrition, diabetes and underlying **cardiorespiratory disease** predispose to pneumonia and are associated with a greatly increased mortality. Patients with **COPD** have impaired mucociliary clearance and organisms of quite low virulence (e.g. *Haemophilus influenzae*) may spread from the bronchi into the peribronchial lung parenchyma causing bronchopneumonia. Mortality from **influenza infection**, either as a cause of primary pneumonia or associated with secondary bacterial pneumonia, is highest in the **elderly**. **Aspiration pneumonia** is likely to occur in patients with impaired swallowing due to oesophageal or neuromuscular disease, or in patients with impaired consciousness (e.g. epileptic fits, anaesthesia).

Pneumonia in the immunocompromised (e.g. patients with human immunodeficiency virus (HIV) infection or receiving immunosuppressive drugs) is a very specific circumstance in which opportunistic infections (e.g. *Pneumocystis carinii*) are common. A particular approach to investigation and treatment is required in these circumstances (see Chapter 8). Patients who have undergone **splenectomy** are particularly vulnerable to pneumococcal pneumonia and septicaemia, and are usually given pneumococcal vaccination and maintained on life-long penicillin prophylaxis.

Environmental and geographical factors

Although in some cases pneumonia arises by aspiration of endogenous infective organisms from the oropharynx, in other cases the patient's environment is the source of infection with the inhalation of infected droplets from **other patients** (e.g. influenza, tuberculosis), from an **animal source** (e.g. *Chlamydia psittaci* from birds, *Coxiella burnetti* from farm animals) or from other **environmental sources** (e.g. *Legionella pneumophila* from contaminated water systems).

Some infections have a particular **geographical distribution** (e.g. histoplasmosis in North America, typhoid in tropical countries) and need to be considered in patients who live in, or have recently visited, these areas. A knowledge of the **local pattern of prevalent infections** and **antibiotic resistance** in a community is important. For example *Mycoplasma pneumoniae* infection particularly occurs in outbreaks about every 4 years and requires treatment with tetracycline or a macrolide (e.g. erythromycin) antibiotic. Although *Streptococcus pneumoniae* in the UK is usually sensitive to penicillin, about 30% of strains isolated in Spain are resistant and this should be borne in mind when choosing initial antibiotic therapy.

Severity of pneumonia

Pneumonia should also be classified according to the severity of the illness. The presence of features indicating severe pneumonia or the occurrence of pneumonia in the context of concomitant illnesses (e.g. chronic cardiorespiratory disease) are important factors in deciding that a patient should be treated **in hospital** rather than **at home**, or in an **intensive therapy unit** (ITU) rather than on a general ward. The features associated with an increased risk of death are shown in Table 6.1.

Clinical features

Patients with pneumonia typically present with **cough, purulent sputum** and **fever**, often accompanied by **pleuritic pain** and **dyspnoea**. There may be a history of a recent upper respiratory tract infection. Diagnosing the site and severity of respiratory tract infection is notoriously difficult and careful assessment combined with good clinical judgement is important. Early review of the situation is crucial in the event of deterioration since the

SEVERE PNEUMONIA

Clinical
Respiratory rate ≥ 30/min
Diastolic blood pressure < 60 mmHg
Age ≥ 60 years
Underlying disease
Confusion
Atrial fibrillation
Multilobar involvement

Laboratory
Serum urea ≥ 7 mmol/L
Serum albumin < 35 g/L
Hypoxaemia $Po_2 \leq 8$ kPa (60 mmHg)
Leucopenia WCC $\leq 4000 \times 10^9$/L
Leucocytosis WCC $\geq 20\,000 \times 10^9$/L
Bacteraemia

WCC, white cell count.

Table 6.1 Indices of severe pneumonia.

severity of the illness is often underestimated by the patient and doctor alike. **Localized chest signs** such as crackles, dullness or bronchial breathing indicate pneumonia rather than bronchitis, for example, but may not always be present. Cyanosis and tachypnoea are features of respiratory failure. Rigors, high fever or prostration suggest septicaemia. Elderly patients, in particular, may present with non-respiratory symptoms such as confusion.

The initial clinical approach focuses on an **assessment of the circumstances and severity** of the illness since these guide decisions as to how and where the patient should be treated. Rather than diagnosing a patient as having a 'chest infection' an effort should be made to use an appropriate descriptive phrase such as: 'a previously fit adult with severe community-acquired pneumonia and suspected septicaemia (rigors, prostration)' or 'probable bronchopneumonia (crackles) and respiratory failure (cyanosis) in a patient with COPD'.

Investigation

Patients with mild pneumonia which responds rapidly to antibiotics are usually treated at home and in this situation investigations don't usually influence management or outcome. Nonetheless, microbiology laboratories will often request that general practitioners send sputum and serology samples from some patients treated in the community so as to be able to alert clinicians to outbreaks of influenza or *Mycoplasma pneumoniae* for example, and to provide information on local patterns of bacterial resistance to antibiotics. More extensive investigations are indicated for patients requiring admission to hospital.

General investigations
• **Chest X-ray** confirms the diagnosis of pneumonia by demonstrating consolidation, detects complications such as lung abscess or empyema, and helps to exclude any underlying disease (e.g. bronchial carcinoma) (Fig. 6.2).
• **Haematology and biochemistry tests**

are useful in assessing the severity of the disease (see Table 6.1).

Further investigations may be indicated if alternative diagnoses are being considered (e.g. ventilation/perfusion scan for pulmonary embolism). Where there is a suspicion of aspiration pneumonia a radiocontrast oesophagogram (e.g. 'Gastrografin swallow') is useful in assessing swallowing problems. Recurrent pneumonia may be an indication of an immunodeficiency state and tests such as measurement of immunoglobulin levels or HIV testing should be performed as appropriate.

Specific investigations
These are aimed at detecting the pathogen causing the pneumonia.
• **Sputum Gram stain** may give a valuable and rapid clue to the responsible organism in an ill patient.
• **Sputum culture** is the main test used to detect bacterial causes of pneumonia but contamination of the sample by oropharyngeal organisms, prior use of antibiotics and inability to produce sputum limit the sensitivity and specificity of the test.
• **Blood cultures** should be performed on all patients admitted to hospital but are positive in only about 15% of cases.
• **Pleural fluid** should be aspirated in all patients with pleural effusions and may yield a causative organism or reveal empyema (see Chapter 17).
• **Antigen detection tests** are available for some pathogens. Pneumococcal antigen may be identified in sputum, urine, pleural fluid or blood and may be positive in cases where prior antibiotics limit the sensitivity of cultures. Direct fluorescent antibody staining may detect *Legionella pneumophila* in bronchoalveolar lavage fluid, and tests for *Legionella* antigen in urine are available in some laboratories.
• **Serological tests** allow a retrospective diagnosis of the infecting organism if a rising titre is found between acute and convalescent samples. This is most useful for some viruses and 'atypical pneumonia' organisms such as *Mycoplasma pneumoniae*.

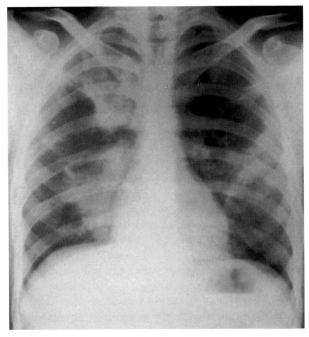

Fig. 6.2 This 60-year-old man was admitted to hospital with a 2-week history of myalgia, headache, dyspnoea and cough without sputum. He was severely ill, cyanosed and delirious with a fever of 39°C, tachycardia of 110/min, respiratory rate 40/min and blood pressure of 110/60 mmHg. Po_2 was 5.7 kPa (43 mmHg), Pco_2 4.9 kPa (37 mmHg), white cell count 4.6×10^9/L and urea 31 mmol/L. He had received amoxycillin for 6 days before admission without improvement. Chest X-ray shows extensive, bilateral multilobar consolidation. He kept birds as a hobby and one of his budgerigars had died recently. The clinical diagnosis of psittacosis was subsequently confirmed by serology tests. He was treated with intravenous fluids, oxygen and tetracycline and recovered fully.

Invasive investigations such as bronchoscopy with bronchoalveolar lavage may be indicated in severe pneumonia and in immunocompromised patients.

Treatment

General

Mild pneumonia in a fit patient can be treated **at home**. Admission to **hospital** is necessary for patients who demonstrate features of severe pneumonia, who have concomitant disease or who do not have adequate family help at home. The severity of the pneumonia should be formally assessed at the time of admission to hospital (see Table 6.1) and elective transfer to an **ITU** should be considered for patients with severe disease.

Sufficient **oxygen** should be given to maintain arterial Po_2 >8 kPa (60 mmHg) and oxygen saturation >90%. Adequate non-sedative **analgesia** (e.g. paracetamol or non-steroidal anti-inflammatory drugs) should be given to control pleuritic pain. **Fluid balance** should be optimized, using intravenous rehydration as required for dehydrated patients. Chest physiotherapy may be beneficial to patients with COPD and copious secretions but is not helpful in patients without underlying lung disease. The patient's general condition, pulse, blood pressure, temperature, respiratory rate and oxygen saturation should be monitored frequently and any deterioration should prompt reassessment of the need for transfer to ITU.

Antibiotic treatment

The initial choice of antibiotics is based upon an assessment of the circumstances and severity of the pneumonia. Treatment is then adjusted in accordance with the patient's response and the results of microbiology investigations. For **community-acquired pneumonia**, *Streptococcus pneumoniae* is the most likely pathogen and **amoxycillin** is an appropriate antibiotic. Where there is a suspicion of 'atypical pneumonia' (e.g. *Mycoplasma pneumoniae*, *Chlamydia psitacci*) addition of a macrolide antibiotic, such as **erythromycin** is required. In **severe pneumonia** the initial antibiotic regimen must cover all likely pathogens and allow for potential antibiotic resistance, and intravenous **cefuroxime and erythromycin** are appropriate. In **hospital-acquired pneumonia**, Gram-negative bacteria are common pathogens, and a combination of an **aminoglycoside** (e.g. gentamicin) and a **third-generation cephalosporin** (e.g. ceftazidime) or an **anti-pseudomonal penicillin** (e.g. azlocillin) is commonly used.

Failure to respond suggests the occurrence of a complication (e.g. empyema), infection with an unusual pathogen (e.g. *Legionella pneumophila*), the presence of antibiotic resistance or incorrect diagnosis (e.g. pulmonary embolism).

Specific pathogens

Pneumococcal pneumonia

Streptococcus pneumoniae is the causative organism in about **60% of community-acquired pneumonias** and in about 10% of hospital-acquired pneumonias. Research studies using tests for pneumococcal antigen suggest that it may account for many cases where no organism is identified. It is a Gram-positive coccus which can cause infections at all levels in the respiratory tract including sinusitis, otitis media, bronchitis and pneumonia. Up to 60% of people carry *Streptococcus pneumoniae* as a **commensal in the nasopharynx** and infection is transmitted in airborne droplets. Nasopharyngeal carriage may progress to infection where there is a breach in the respiratory tract defences, and smoking and viral infections are important factors disrupting surface defence mechanisms. There are many **different serotypes which vary in their virulence**, but virulent stains can render a previously fit and healthy person critically ill within a few hours. Pneumococcal sepsis in asplenic patients (e.g. postsplenectomy) is severe with a high mortality, such that these patients are usually given pneumococcal vaccination and long-term prophylactic phenoxymethylpenicillin 500 mg b.d. *Streptococcus pneumoniae* is usually **sensitive to penicillin antibiotics** (e.g. amoxycillin or benzyl penicillin) but antibiotic **resistance is an emerging problem** particularly in certain countries such as Spain, where about 30% of isolates are resistant, so that it is necessary to give broad antibiotic cover to a patient who has acquired pneumonia in a country with a high prevalence of antibiotic-resistant pneumococcus. **Pneumococcal vaccine** is recommended for patients with chronic lung disease, diabetes, renal, and cardiac disease and for patients who are asplenic or immunodeficient (e.g. hypogammaglobulinaemia, HIV).

Haemophilus influenzae pneumonia

Haemophilus influenzae is a **Gram-negative bacillus**. Virulent strains are encapsulated and divided into six serological types. *Haemophilus influenzae* type b is a virulent encapsulated form which causes **epiglottitis, bacteraemia, meningitis** and **pneumonia**. *Haemophilus influenzae* type b (Hib) vaccine is given to children to reduce the risk of meningitis and this vaccine also provides protection against epiglottitis. However, it is the less virulent form of the organism — **non-typeable unencapsulated *Haemophilus influenzae*** — which is a common cause of respiratory tract infection, predominantly where there has been damage to the bronchial mucosa by smoking or viral infection. *Haemophilus influenzae* often forms part of the normal pharyngeal flora. Deficient mucociliary clearance in patients with smoking-induced chronic bronchitis facilitates spread of the organism to the lower respiratory tract, where it gives rise to **exacerbations of COPD**. Spread of infection into the lung parenchyma causes **bronchopneumoni**a. It is usually treated with **amoxycillin** but about 10% of strains are resistant and alternative antibiotics include co-amoxiclav (amoxycillin with clavulanic acid), trimethoprim, and cefixime.

Staphylococcal pneumonia

Staphylococcus aureus is a **Gram-positive coccus** which forms clusters resembling a bunch of grapes. Although it is a relatively uncommon cause of either community-acquired or hospital-acquired pneumonia it may produce a very **severe illness with a high mortality**. It particularly occurs as a **sequel to influenza** so that anti-staphylococcal antibiotics should be given to patients who develop pneumonia after influenza. Infection may also reach the lungs via the blood stream when staphylococcal bacteraemia arises from intravenous cannulae in hospitalized patients or from intravenous drug misuse, for example. The production of toxins may cause tissue necrosis with cavitation, pneumatocele formation and pneumothoraces. The standard treatment is with β-lactamase-resistant penicillins such as **flucloxacillin**.

Klebsiella pneumonia

Klebsiella pneumoniae is a **Gram-negative organism** which generally causes pneumonia only in **patients who have impaired resistance** to infection (e.g. **alcohol misuse, malnutrition, diabetes**) or **underlying lung disease** (e.g. bronchiectasis). It often produces severe infection with destruction of lung tissue, **cavitation** and **abscess formation**. Treatment requires attention to the underlying disease state and prolonged antibiotic therapy,

guided by the results of microbiology culture and sensitivity. Often a combination of a **third-generation cephalosporin** (e.g. ceftazidime) and an **aminoglycoside** (e.g. gentamicin) is appropriate.

Pseudomonas aeruginosa pneumonia

Pseudomonas aeruginosa is a **Gram-negative bacillus** which is a common cause of **pneumonia in hospitalized patients**, particularly those with neutropenia and those receiving endotracheal ventilation in ITU. It is usually treated with a combination of an aminoglycoside (e.g. gentamicin) and a third-generation cephalosporin (e.g. ceftazidime) or **antipseudomonal penicillin** (e.g. azlocillin).

Atypical pneumonia

'Atypical pneumonia' is an imprecise term which is sometimes used in clinical practice to refer to pneumonia caused by *Mycoplasma pneumoniae*, chlamydial organisms, and *Legionella pneumophila*. Characteristically these organisms are **not sensitive to penicillins** and require treatment with **tetracycline or macrolide (e.g. erythromycin)** antibiotics. These organisms are **difficult to culture** in the laboratory and the diagnosis is often made retrospectively by demonstrating a rising antibody titre on serological tests.

Mycoplasma pneumonia

Mycoplasma pneumoniae is a small, free-living organism, which does not have a rigid cell wall and which is therefore not susceptible to antibiotics such as penicillin which act on bacterial cell walls. Infection is transmitted from person to person by infected respiratory droplets. It **particularly affects children and young adults** although any age group may be affected. Infection typically occurs in **outbreaks every 4 years** and spreads throughout families, schools and colleges. *Mycoplasma pneumoniae* typically causes an initial upper respiratory tract infection with pharyngitis, sinusitis and otitis, followed by pneumonia in about 30% of cases. A variety of **extrapulmonary syndromes** may occur and may be related to immune responses to infection. These include lymphocytic meningoencephalitis, cerebellar ataxia, peripheral neuropathy, rashes, arthralgia, splenomegaly and hepatitis. **Cold agglutinins** to type O red cells are often present and haemolytic anaemia may occur. *Mycoplasma pneumoniae* causes significant protracted morbidity but is rarely life threatening.

Chlamydial respiratory infections

There are three chlamydial species which cause respiratory disease:
• *Chlamydia psittaci* is primarily an infection of **birds** which is transmitted to humans as a **zoonosis** (a disease contracted from animals) by inhalation of contaminated droplets. Psittacosis or ornithosis is the name given to the resultant illness which is often severe and characterized by high fever, headache, delirium, a macular rash and severe pneumonia.
• *Chlamydia pneumoniae* was identified as a respiratory pathogen in 1986. Infection is confined to **humans** and there is no avian or animal reservoir of infection. Infection with this organism is extremely common in all age groups and spreads directly from **person to person**, with **outbreaks occurring in families, schools and colleges**. It typically produces upper respiratory disease including pharyngitis, otitis and sinusitis but may also cause pneumonia which is usually mild.
• *Chlamydia trachomatis* is a common cause of sexually transmitted genital tract infection and **infants** may acquire respiratory tract infection with this organism from their mother's genital tract during birth.

Legionella pneumonia

Legionella pneumophila is a **Gram-negative bacillus** which is widely distributed in nature in **water**. The organism was first identified in 1976 when an outbreak of severe pneumonia affected delegates at a convention of the American Legion, who contracted infection from a contaminated humidifier system (**Legionnaires' disease**). In sporadic cases there is often no apparent source for the infection. Sometimes infection can be traced back to a **contaminated water system** such as a shower in a hotel bedroom. Epidemics of infection may occur from a common source such as a contaminated humidification plant, water storage tanks or heating circuits. Infection does not spread from patient to patient. *Legionella pneumophila* typically causes a **severe pneumonia** with prostration, confusion, diarrhoea, abdominal pain and respiratory failure, with an associated high mortality. Direct fluorescent antibody staining may detect the organism in bronchoalveolar lavage fluid, and tests to detect *Legionella* antigen in urine are available, and allow rapid diagnosis. A combination of erythromycin and rifampicin is often used to treat severe *Legionella* pneumonia.

Further reading

American Thoracic Society. Hospital-acquired pneumonia in adults: diagnosis, assessment of severity, initial antimicrobial therapy, and preventative strategies. *Am J Respir Crit Care Med* 1995; **153**: 1711–25.

Bourke SJ. Chlamydial respiratory infections. *BMJ* 1993; **306**: 1219–20.

British Thoracic Society. Guidelines for the management of community-acquired pneumonia in adults admitted to hospital. *Br J Hosp Med* 1993; **49**: 346–50.

Obaro SK, Monteil MA, Henderson DC. The pneumococcal problem. *BMJ* 1996; **312**: 1521–5.

Roig J, Domingo C, Morera J. Legionnaires' Disease. *Chest* 1994; **105**: 1817–24.

CHAPTER 7

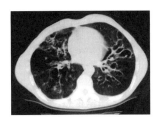

Tuberculosis

Tuberculosis is an infection due to *Mycobacterium tuberculosis* which may affect any part of the body but most commonly affects the lungs.

Epidemiology

The World Health Organization estimates that **1.72 billion people (one-third of the world's population) have latent infection with *Mycobacterium tuberculosis*, 15–20 million people have active infection** and **3 million deaths occur each year** from tuberculosis (95% in the developing world). One hundred years ago in the UK more than 30 000 people died from tuberculosis each year (about the same as for lung cancer at present). Mortality and notification rates declined steadily from 1900 onwards due to improvement in nutritional and social factors, with a sharper decline occurring from the late 1940s onwards due to the introduction of effective treatment. Overall the decline in notification rates has levelled off over the last decade, with some areas noting small increases (Fig. 7.1). Notification rates in the UK are 20–30 times higher in people of Indian origin than in the indigenous white population. About 33% of all cases in the UK occur in those of Indian origin (80% of these are under 55 years of age) with the highest rates occurring in the early years after immigration. About 60% of cases occur in the white population (more than 50% of these

are over 55 years of age). Infection may have been contracted in childhood and lain dormant for years before reactivating. Factors which reduce resistance and precipitate reactivation include ageing, alcohol misuse, poor nutrition, debility from other diseases, use of immuno-suppressive drug therapy, and co-infection with human immunodeficiency virus (HIV). In the UK, overlap between the population with HIV infection (mainly young white men) and the population with tuberculosis (mainly older white people and younger immigrants from the Indian subcontinent) is limited so that only 5% of patients with acquired immune deficiency syndrome (AIDS) have tuberculosis and about 2% of patients with tuberculosis are identified as having HIV infection. However, **4.5 million people worldwide are estimated to be co-infected with HIV and tuberculosis** (98% in developing countries).

Clinical course (Fig. 7.2)

The clinical course of tuberculosis often evolves over many years and represents a complex interaction between the infecting organism (*Mycobacterium tuberculosis*) and the person's specific immune response and non-specific resistance to infection. Traditional descriptions of tuberculosis divide the disease into two main patterns, **primary** and **post-primary** tuberculosis, although these are

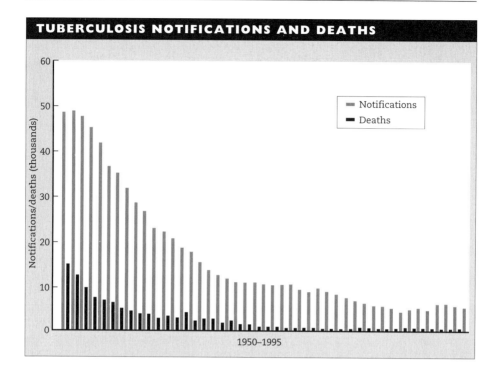

TUBERCULOSIS NOTIFICATIONS AND DEATHS

Fig. 7.1 Notifications of tuberculosis and deaths in England and Wales, 1950–1995. Notifications of tuberculosis have declined from about 50 000 in 1950 to 5000 in 1987, since when notifications have plateaued. (Reproduced with permission from *The Prevention and Control of Tuberculosis in the United Kingdom,* Department of Health, 1996.)

mainly based upon the characteristic evolution of the disease in the days before effective chemotherapy.

Primary tuberculosis

Primary tuberculosis is the pattern of disease seen with **first infection** in a person (often a child) **without specific immunity** to tuberculosis. Infection is acquired by inhalation of organisms from an infected individual, and the initial lesion typically develops in the peripheral, subpleural, region of the lung followed by a reaction in the hilar lymph nodes. The **primary complex** appears on chest X-ray as a peripheral area of consolidation (Gohn focus) and hilar adenopathy. Occasionally, erythema nodosum develops at this stage. An immune response develops, the tuberculin test becomes positive and **healing** often takes place. This stage of the disease is often asymptomatic but may leave calcified nodules on chest X-rays representing the healed primary focus. Active **progression** of first infection may occur. Bronchial spread of infection may cause progressive consolidation and cavitation of the lung parenchyma, and pleural effusions may develop. Lymphatic spread of infection may cause progressive lymph node enlargement, which in children may compress bronchi with obstruction, distal consolidation and the development of collapse and bronchiectasis. Bronchiectasis of the middle lobe is a very typical outcome of hilar node involvement by tuberculosis in childhood. Haematogenous spread of infection results in early generalization of disease which may cause miliary tuberculosis, and the lethal complication of tuberculous meningitis (par-

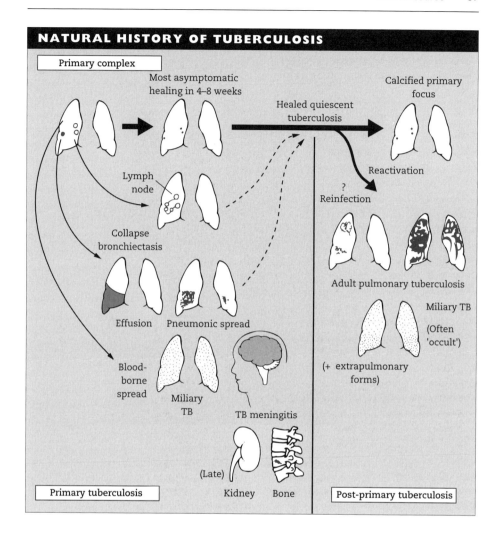

NATURAL HISTORY OF TUBERCULOSIS

Primary complex

Most asymptomatic
healing in 4–8 weeks

Calcified primary
focus

Healed quiescent
tuberculosis

Reactivation

Lymph
node

?
Reinfection

Collapse
bronchiectasis

Adult pulmonary tuberculosis

Effusion   Pneumonic spread

Miliary TB

(Often
'occult')

Blood-
borne
spread

Miliary
TB

TB meningitis

(+ extrapulmonary
forms)

(Late)

Kidney   Bone

Primary tuberculosis

Post-primary tuberculosis

Fig. 7.2 Summary of the natural history of tuberculosis.

ticularly in young children). Infection spread during this initial illness may lie **dormant** in any organ of the body (e.g. bone, kidneys) for many years only to **reactivate** many years later.

Post-primary tuberculosis

Post-primary tuberculosis is the **pattern of disease seen after the development of specific immunity**. It may occur following direct progression of the initial infection or result from endogenous **reactivation** of infection or from exogenous **re-infection** (inhalation of *Mycobacterium tuberculosis* from another infected individual) in a patient who has had previous contact with the organism and has developed a degree of specific immunity. Reactivation particularly occurs in old age and in circumstances (e.g. illness, alcohol misuse, immunosuppressive drug treatment) where immunocompetence is impaired. The lungs are the most usual site of post-primary disease and the apices of the lungs are the commonest pulmonary site.

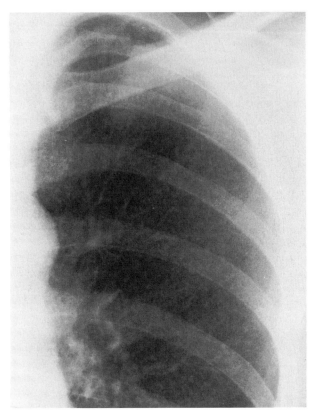

Fig. 7.3 This 24-year-old man presented with malaise, fever and weight loss without any respiratory symptoms. Six months previously he had immigrated to the UK from Bangladesh. X-ray shows multiple 1–2 mm nodules throughout both lungs characteristic of miliary tuberculosis. Sputum and bronchoalveolar lavage did not show acid- and alcohol-fast bacilli (AAFB). Transbronchial biopsies, however, showed caseating granulomas characteristic of tuberculosis. His symptoms resolved and the chest X-ray appearances returned to normal after 6 months of anti-tuberculosis chemotherapy.

Diagnosis

Clinical features

Definitive diagnosis requires identification of *Mycobacterium tuberculosis* because the clinical features of the disease are non-specific. The most typical **chest symptoms** are persistent cough, sputum production and haemoptysis. **Systemic symptoms** include fever, night sweats, anorexia and weight loss. A range of **chest X-ray** abnormalities occur (Figs 7.3 and 7.4). Cavitating apical lesions are characteristic of tuberculosis but such lesions may also be caused by lung cancer. Irregular mottled shadowing (particularly of the lung apices) streaky fibrosis, calcified granuloma, miliary mottling, pleural effusions and hilar gland enlargement may all be features of tuberculosis.

Diagnosis depends on the doctor having a high level of awareness of the many presentations of tuberculosis and undertaking appropriate investigations (e.g. sputum **acid- and alcohol-fast bacilli** (AAFB) staining and culture for tuberculosis) in patients with persistent chest symptoms or abnormal X-rays. A high index of suspicion is required in assess-

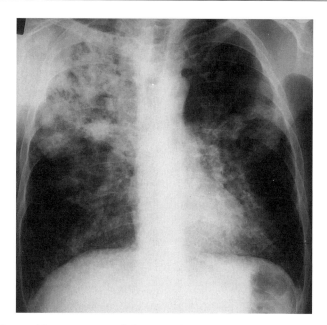

Fig. 7.4 This 68-year-old man was persuaded to consult a doctor because of a 6-month history of cough, haemoptysis, night sweats and weight loss. He suffered from alcoholism and lived in a hostel for homeless men. His chest X-ray shows cavitating consolidation throughout the right upper lobe with further areas of consolidation in the left upper and right lower lobes. Sputum acid- and alcohol-fast bacilli (AAFB) stains were positive and cultures yielded *Mycobacterium* *tuberculosis* sensitive to standard drugs. He was treated with directly observed anti-tuberculosis therapy. Six of 38 residents of the hostel were found to have active tuberculosis. DNA fingerprinting techniques showed that this cluster of six cases was due to three different strains of *Mycobacterium tuberculosis* arising as a result of both reactivation of latent tuberculosis in debilitated elderly men and spread of infection within the hostel.

ing patients who have recently immigrated from a high prevalence area (e.g. Indian subcontinent), and in patients at risk for reactivation of infection because of factors which lower their resistance (age, alcohol misuse, debilitating disease, use of immunosuppressive drugs).

Although tuberculosis most commonly affects the lungs, **any organ in the body may be involved** and the diagnosis needs to be considered in patients with a **pyrexia of unknown origin** and patients with a variety of indolent chronic lesions (e.g. in bone, kidney or lymph nodes). The term **miliary tuberculosis** refers to a situation where there has been widespread haematogenous dissemination of tuberculosis, usually with multiple (millet-seed size) nodules evident on chest X-ray. Chest symptoms are often minimal and typically the patient is ill and pyrexial with anaemia and weight loss.

Laboratory diagnosis

Identification of *Mycobacterium tuberculosis* by laboratory tests may take some time and anti-tuberculosis treatment may have to be commenced based on clinical and radiological features whilst awaiting the results of laboratory tests. Once the diagnosis is suspected, repeated **sputum** samples should be examined by the **Ziehl–Neelsen** (ZN) method looking for AAFB which appear as red rods on a blue background. **Sputum cultures** require special media (e.g. Löwenstein–Jensen medium) and the tubercle bacillus grows slowly taking 4–7 weeks to give a positive culture and a further 3 weeks for the *in vitro* testing of antibiotic sensitivity. **Biopsy** of an affected site (e.g. pleura, lymph node, liver, bone marrow) may show the characteristic features of **caseating granuloma** (central cheesy necrosis of a lesion formed by macrophages, lymphocytes and epithelial cells). Biopsy specimens should also be submitted for mycobacterial cultures. Newer techniques are being developed to improve the speed, sensitivity and specificity of the laboratory diagnosis of tuberculosis. The **Bactec radiometric system**, for example, uses a liquid medium containing a radioactively labelled ^{14}C-labelled substance which releases $^{14}CO_2$ when metabolized, and detection of this reflects the growth of *Mycobacterium tuberculosis*. DNA techniques using the **polymerase chain reaction** are being developed and may, for example, prove useful in detecting evidence of infection in cerebrospinal fluid in tuberculous meningitis. **DNA finger-print techniques make it possible to distinguish different strains of Mycobacterium tuberculosis**. This can give useful insights into the likely sources and spread of infection and help assess the relative contribution of newly acquired and reactivated infection in different populations.

Treatment (Table 7.1)

Before effective antibiotics became available in the late 1940s, about 50% of patients with sputum-positive tuberculosis died of the disease. Patients were admitted to sanatoria for bed rest, 'sunshine and fresh air' therapy and nutritional support in an attempt to enhance their own resistance to the disease. When large tuberculous cavities developed in the lungs attempts were made to collapse the cavities by inducing an artificial pneumothorax, crushing the phrenic nerve, instilling various materials outside the pleura to compress the lung (plombage) or performing thoracoplasty, whereby the ribs were excised and the lung compressed against the mediastinum. In the late 1940s **streptomycin** and **para-amino salicylic acid** (PAS) were introduced into clinical practice and the outlook for patients with tuberculosis was revolutionized. It soon became apparent that treatment had to be **prolonged** and **combinations** of antibiotics had to be used because of the capacity of the tubercle bacillus to lie dormant in lesions for

TUBERCULOSIS TREATMENT

Drug	Dose		Duration	Adverse effects
	Children	Adult		
Isoniazid	10 mg/kg	300 mg	6 months	Hepatitis, neuropathy
Rifampicin	10 mg/kg	<50 kg 450 mg	6 months	Hepatitis, rashes
		≥50 kg 600 mg		enzyme induction
Pyrazinamide	35 mg/kg	<50 kg 1.5 g	Initial	Hepatitis, rashes
		≥50 kg 2.0 g	2 months	elevated uric acid

- 6 months of rifampicin and isoniazid, with pyrazinamide for first 2 months
- Monitor treatment meticulously (e.g. monthly review)
- Check compliance
- Use directly observed therapy if problems with compliance
- Notify the diagnosis to Public Health Authorities
- Contact tracing of close family contacts

Table 7.1 Treatment of tuberculosis.

long periods and to develop resistance to antibiotics.

The current standard treatment of tuberculosis consists of **6 months** of **rifampicin** and **isoniazid**, supplemented by **pyrazinamide** for the first 2 months. All drugs are usually given in a single daily dose. Rifampicin and isoniazid are bactericidal drugs which kill extracellular bacilli which are actively metabolizing. Both rifampicin and pyrazinamide are effective against intracellular bacilli, within macrophages. Prolonged treatment is needed to eradicate bacilli lying dormant. The use of the combination of drugs also prevents the emergence of resistance from the small number of bacilli which are naturally resistant to any one of the antibiotics. Meticulous **supervision** of treatment is essential and patients should be seen at least monthly for prescription of medication, checking of **compliance** with treatment and monitoring for side-effects (e.g. liver function tests). Errors in the prescription of medication or failure of the patient to comply with treatment may have disastrous consequences with the emergence of resistant organisms. **Directly observed therapy** should be instituted for patients who have difficulty complying with treatment, whereby the patient is observed to ensure that he or she swallows the medication. Sometimes this can be achieved by giving high doses of the anti-tuberculosis medication three times per week with the patient attending a hospital or general practice clinic to be given the medication under the supervision of a doctor or nurse. Flexible strategies are required to ensure compliance of patients with social (e.g. homelessness) or psychological (e.g. alcohol misuse, mental illness) problems and there is an important role for community health workers or trained lay persons in these circumstances.

At present, **drug-resistant tuberculosis** is rare in the initial treatment of white patients in the UK. About 6% of patients from the Indian subcontinent have tuberculosis which is resistant to isoniazid, and in this situation an additional drug, such as **ethambutol**, is added to their treatment regimen. **Multi-drug-resistant tuberculosis** results from inadequate previous treatment. The development of resistant organisms in a patient failing to comply with treatment may make the tuberculosis very difficult to treat, and such a patient poses a risk to public health since he or she may infect others with drug-resistant tuberculosis. Some outbreaks of multi-drug-resistant tuberculosis have occurred in prisons and hospitals with high mortality rates.

The most dangerous of the **adverse reactions** to anti-tuberculosis treatment is **hepatotoxicity**, and patients should be advised to stop treatment and report for medical advice if they develop fever, vomiting, malaise or jaundice. Isoniazid, rifampicin and pyrazinamide may all cause hepatitis and allergic reactions such as **rashes**. Isoniazid may cause a **peripheral neuropathy** and this is preventable by pyridoxine 10 mg/day, which is given routinely to those at risk of neuropathy (e.g. patients with diabetes or alcohol misuse). Intermittent rifampicin may cause 'flu like' symptoms, and the **induction of microsomal hepatic enzymes** reduces the serum half-life of drugs such as warfarin, steroids, phenytoin and oestrogen contraceptives so that patients may need adjustment in dosage of medications and may need to use alternative contraceptive measures. Rifampicin produces a reddish discolouration of urine (which may be used to monitor compliance) and may cause staining of soft contact lenses. Pyrazinamide sometimes causes initial facial flushing, and may cause an **elevation of uric acid levels** with arthralgia. Ethambutol causes a dose-related **optic neuropathy**, which is rare at doses below 15 mg/kg/day. Patients should be warned to stop the drug if visual symptoms occur, and the drug should be avoided if possible in patients with impaired renal function or pre-existing visual problems.

Tuberculin testing (Fig. 7.5)

Hypersensitivity to the tubercle bacillus can be

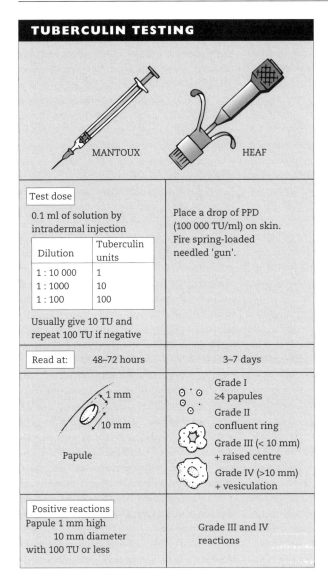

TUBERCULIN TESTING

MANTOUX   HEAF

Test dose	
0.1 ml of solution by intradermal injection	Place a drop of PPD (100 000 TU/ml) on skin. Fire spring-loaded needled 'gun'.

Dilution	Tuberculin units
1 : 10 000	1
1 : 1000	10
1 : 100	100

Usually give 10 TU and repeat 100 TU if negative

Read at:	48–72 hours	3–7 days

1 mm
10 mm
Papule

Grade I
≥4 papules
Grade II
confluent ring
Grade III (< 10 mm)
+ raised centre
Grade IV (>10 mm)
+ vesiculation

Positive reactions	
Papule 1 mm high 10 mm diameter with 100 TU or less	Grade III and IV reactions

Fig. 7.5 Tuberculin testing.

detected by the intradermal injection of a purified protein derivative (PPD) of the organism. The response is of the type IV cell-mediated variety and results in a raised area of induration and reddening of the skin. In the **Mantoux test** 0.1 ml of tuberculin solution is injected intradermally (not subcutaneously) and the test is read at 48–72 hours. A positive result is indicated by redness and induration at least 10 mm in diameter. If active tuberculosis is suspected the lowest dilution may be used initially to prevent a severe reaction, and higher concentrations used if there is no reaction. The **Heaf test** is performed with a spring-loaded needled 'gun'. A drop of undiluted PPD (100 000 TU/ml) is placed on the volar surface of the forearm and the 'gun' is used to puncture through the PPD solution. The reaction is graded from I to IV according to the formation of papules and the extent of induration. A positive tuberculin test indicates the presence of hypersensitivity to tuberculin resulting from either previous infection with tubercle bacillus or from bacillus Calmette–Guérin (BCG) vaccination. A weak reaction may be non-specific and indicate contact with other non-tuberculous environmental mycobacteria. A strongly positive test in a child who has not received BCG vaccination is likely to indicate primary infection. If there is evidence of active disease, full anti-tuberculosis treatment is required; if there is no evidence of active disease chemoprophylaxis is advisable. A source amongst adult contacts of the child must be carefully sought. A negative tuberculin test makes active tuberculosis unlikely and indicates a lack of immunity so that BCG vaccination is recommended.

Control

Treating active disease
Prompt **identification** and **treatment** of patients with active tuberculosis limits the spread of infection. Sputum-positive patients (AAFB positive) should be considered as potentially infectious until they have completed 2 weeks of treatment. The patient's family will already have been exposed to the risk of infection so that segregation of the patient from contact with his or her family at the time of diagnosis is not useful, and most patients can be treated as outpatients. Where patients with suspected or confirmed tuberculosis are admitted to hospital they should be kept in a single room. Particular care is required if the patient has multi-drug-resistant tuberculosis and these patients should be treated in isolation rooms vented to the outside to prevent transmission of infection to other patients or health-care workers.

Contact tracing
When a diagnosis of tuberculosis is made there is a statutory requirement in the UK for the doctor to **notify** the patient to the public health authorities who are then responsible for

undertaking **screening of contacts**. The index patient may have acquired infection from, or transmitted infection to, someone in his or her close environment. It is usual to limit contact tracing to household contacts and to close friends sharing a similar level of contact with the index patient. If initial investigations reveal a large number of contacts with tuberculosis, consideration should be given to widening the circle of contacts who are offered screening. About 10% of close contacts of smear-positive cases are found to have active disease.

Screening of contacts consists of a combination of **chest X-ray, tuberculin testing** (Heaf or Mantoux testing) and checking of **BCG status**. The precise protocol used depends on an assessment of the diagnostic yield of the screening procedure in particular circumstances. Most cases of active tuberculosis are found at the first clinic visit in unvaccinated close contacts of smear-positive disease. Adults should have a chest X-ray performed. In contacts of smear-negative patients this is all that is required. Contacts of smear-positive patients are at greater risk of having inhaled tubercle bacilli and may take weeks or months to develop signs of disease so that follow-up X-rays at 3 and 12 months are advisable. Contacts are often well motivated to attend for initial screening but are often reluctant to return for prolonged follow-up. If the contact has not had **BCG vaccination** a tuberculin test is performed and if this is negative vaccination is recommended. For children a tuberculin test is the usual initial screening test. Children with a strongly positive tuberculin test should have a chest X-ray. A strongly positive tuberculin test (e.g. Heaf grade III or IV) with a normal chest X-ray suggests that the child has been infected with tubercle bacillus, has not developed active disease but remains at risk of doing so in the future. The risk of future activation of such latent infection is reduced by **chemoprophylaxis** which consists of treatment for 6 months with isoniazid alone, or for 3 months with isoniazid and rifampicin. Those with a negative tuberculin test should have it repeated 6 weeks later (to ensure they are not in the process of developing immunity to recently acquired infection), and if they remain tuberculin negative BCG vaccination is advisable. Although most cases of active disease are detected at the initial screening visit, more prolonged follow-up of Asian contacts may be advisable since studies indicate a small but significant late pick-up rate in this group.

Screening of immigrants

Immigrants from areas with a high prevalence of tuberculosis (e.g. Indian subcontinent) should be screened for tuberculosis on arrival in a country of low-prevalence such as the UK. Adults should have a chest X-ray and children should have a tuberculin test. Thereafter the procedure is as for close contacts with treatment of active disease, chemoprophylaxis of latent infection, or BCG vaccination as appropriate.

BCG vaccination

BCG is a live attenuated strain of tuberculosis which **provides about 75% protection against tuberculosis for about 15 years**. It is given by intradermal injection (not subcutaneous injection) and produces a local skin reaction. It is currently given to children aged 13 years in the UK and to younger children in contact with known cases of tuberculosis. The need for routine BCG vaccination in the UK has been questioned but the BCG vaccination procedure is being continued at present because of the recent increase in tuberculosis in some countries and the cessation of the decline in notifications in the UK.

Opportunistic mycobacteria (atypical mycobacteria)

There are a number of other mycobacteria which can cause pulmonary disease and which do not belong to the Mycobacterium tuberculosis complex. These are called 'atypical' or 'oppor-

tunistic' mycobacteria and the most common of these are **Mycobacterium kansasii**, **Mycobacterium avium-intracellulare complex**, **Mycobacterium malmoense** and **Mycobacterium xenopi**. They are widespread in nature and can be found in water and soil so that sometimes contamination of clinical specimens occurs from environmental sources. They act as low-grade pathogens which do not pose a risk to normal individuals. Infections occur in patients with impaired immunity, e.g. AIDS (see Chapter 8) or in those with severely damaged lungs (e.g. advanced emphysema or lung cavities from previous Mycobacterium tuberculosis infection). They are often associated with chronic symptoms such as cough, sputum production, haemoptysis and weight loss. Diagnosis is made on the basis of their characteristics on laboratory culture tests. Treatment is often difficult requiring prolonged (e.g. 2 years) treatment with rifampicin and ethambutol since these organisms often show resistance to some standard anti-tuberculosis antibiotics. Some more recently developed antibiotics, e.g. clarithromycin or ciprofloxacin, may be useful in treatment. These organisms are low-grade pathogens and do not pose a threat to contacts of infected patients so that there is no need for contact tracing procedures.

Further reading

Morse DI. Directly observed therapy for tuberculosis. BMJ 1996; **312**: 719–20.

Ormerod LP. Chemotherapy and management of tuberculosis in the United Kingdom. British Thoracic Society guidelines. Thorax 1990; **45**: 403–8.

Skinner C. Control and prevention of tuberculosis in the United Kingdom. Thorax 1994; **49**: 1193–200.

Sudre P, Dam G, Kochi A. Tuberculosis: a global overview of the situation today. Bull WHO 1992; **70**: 149–59.

Van Soolingen D, Hermans PWM. Epidemiology of tuberculosis by DNA fingerprinting. Eur Respir J 1995; **8** (suppl. 20): 649–56.

CHAPTER 8

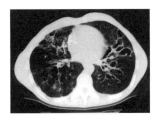

Respiratory Disease in AIDS and Immunocompromised Patients

Acquired immune deficiency syndrome

Acquired immune deficiency syndrome (AIDS) was first recognized in 1981 when clusters of cases of Kaposi's sarcoma and *Pneumocystis carinii* pneumonia (PCP) were found among homosexual men in the USA. Human immunodeficiency virus (HIV) type 1 was identified as the cause of AIDS in 1983. Infection is transmitted by **sexual intercourse**, by **perinatal transmission** and by exposure to **infected blood**.

Epidemiology
Global
It is estimated that since the first case of AIDS was recognized 15 years ago, about 5 million people have died from AIDS, and that about 24 million adults and 1.5 million children have been infected with HIV. About two-thirds of cases have been in Africa where **heterosexual intercourse** is the main mode of transmission and where as many women as men are infected. There is a high rate of **perinatal transmission** of infection to babies born of infected mothers by maternofetal transfer *in utero*, during delivery or by breast feeding. Globally the pandemic is still escalating, particularly in sub-Saharan Africa and South-East Asia, with an estimated 10000 new infections occurring each day.

UK
In the UK about 27000 people are infected with HIV. About 60% of these are **homosexual** or **bisexual** men, 20% are **intravenous drug users** and 20% were infected through **heterosexual intercourse**. The proportion of infections directly attributed to homosexual transmission seems to be decreasing as 'safe sex' practices (e.g. use of condoms) are adopted by homosexual men. The prevalence of infection in intravenous drug users and in heterosexual partners of infected persons seems to be increasing. The treatment of **haemophiliacs** with Factor VIII concentrates derived from large numbers of donors led to a high incidence of HIV infection. Routine testing for HIV in donated blood in the developed countries has stopped transmission of infection in blood products and transfusions.

Human immunodeficiency virus infection

HIV is a retrovirus which has a high affinity for the CD_4 molecule of T lymphocytes. After **binding to the CD_4 receptor** the virus penetrates the cell wall and initiates a cycle of **viral replication** within the cell. The replication of retroviruses is driven by the enzyme **reverse transcriptase** which translates the single-stranded viral RNA back to double-stranded

DNA—hence the term 'retro' or 'reverse'. The viral DNA is **integrated** into the genome of the cell by the viral enzyme, integrase, and this provirus is then propagated in subsequent generations after each round of cell division. The provirus may remain silent during the cell's lifetime or be **transcribed**, producing new viral particles which form buds on the cell membrane. The transcription of the provirus is controlled by various proteins derived from the virus itself and from the host cell. On death of the T cell the virus is released and taken up by new cells, **propagating** infection further. HIV infection results in a progressive fall in the number and function of CD$_4$ T lymphocytes. The pace at which immunodeficiency develops and the susceptibility to opportunistic infections is reflected in the **CD$_4$ lymphocyte count**. It is possible to measure the HIV replication rate by measuring plasma concentrations of HIV RNA, and this is often referred to as the '**viral load**'.

The average time from initial infection with HIV to the development of AIDS is about 10–12 years. After primary infection with HIV there is an asymptomatic period of about 4 weeks. Then many patients will suffer a 2–3-week **seroconversion illness** which resembles glandular fever with malaise, arthralgia, lymphadenopathy, headache, rashes and fever. This phase is associated with high levels of viraemia, and towards the end of this phase antibodies to HIV are detectable. The virus then becomes mainly localized in lymphoid tissue and the disease enters a chronic symptomless phase. **Persistent generalized lymphadenopathy** may develop with enlarged nodes in more than one site persisting for more than 3 months. Some patients develop symptoms such as malaise, weight loss and fevers which are due to HIV infection but not the consequence of opportunistic infections. **AIDS** is diagnosed when an HIV-seropositive patient develops certain major opportunistic infections (e.g. *Pneumocystis carinii* pneumonia, *Mycobacterium avium-intracellulare*) or defined malignancies (e.g. Kaposi's sarcoma, non-Hodgkin's lymphoma).

Anti-retroviral treatments
(Table 8.1)

Anti-retroviral treatments aim to produce benefit to patients by disrupting key stages in the HIV replication cycle. At present the two main classes of drugs available are **reverse transcriptase inhibitors**, which inhibit the incorporation of viral genetic material into the T-cell genome by inhibiting the translation of viral RNA back to DNA, and **proteinase inhibitors**, which inhibit the viral

ANTI-RETROVIRAL DRUGS

Mode of action	Drug	Adverse effects
Reverse transcriptase inhibitors (inhibit translation of HIV RNA back to DNA for incorporation into T-cell genome)	Zidovudine (AZT) Didanosine (ddI) Zalcitabine (ddC) Lamivudine (3TC) Stavudine (d4T) Nevirapine	Marrow suppression, nausea Pancreatitis Neuropathy, nausea Pancreatitis Neuropathy Rash
Proteinase inhibitors (inhibit the translation of HIV provirus from the T-cell genome)	Indinavir Ritonavir Saquinavir	Renal calculi Neuropathy, nausea Headache

Table 8.1 Anti-retroviral drugs.

proteinases which control the translation of HIV provirus from the T-cell genome. Other drugs such as integrase inhibitors are being developed.

Initial studies using zidovudine (AZT) monotherapy gave disappointing results and highlighted the potential for the development of drug resistance. Dual therapy, using two reverse transcriptase inhibitors (e.g. zidovudine and didanosine) gave better results and current attempts at triple therapy, adding a proteinase inhibitor (e.g. indinavir), are promising. Measurement of 'viral load' (e.g. plasma HIV RNA) and CD_4 T-lymphocyte counts are useful in monitoring the progression of the disease and the effects of treatment, and there is increasing evidence that giving intensive anti-retroviral combination therapy when a high viral load is present improves survival and delays progression of the disease. Anti-retroviral drugs have significant toxicities and are expensive (particularly when most patients with HIV are in developing countries), and long-term efficacy is uncertain. The optimum use of anti-retroviral drugs is the subject of intense research. There are many analogies with the development of anti-tuberculous drugs in the 1940s.

Pulmonary complications of human immunodeficiency virus infection (Table 8.2)

Although CD_4 T lymphocytes are the main target of HIV infection, the virus also infects other cells in the body including pulmonary macrophages. A **lymphocytic alveolitis** and **impaired gas diffusion** (reduced transfer factor for carbon monoxide) are found even in asymptomatic patients who do not have evidence of opportunistic infections. Early in the course of HIV infection **asthma** and **atopic disease** seem to be more common, possibly because of an increase in circulating IgE levels as part of the complex immune response to HIV infection. The occurrence of various infections reflects the CD_4 T-lymphocyte count and depends on the patient's previous and current exposure to pathogens (e.g. reactivation of previous tuberculosis or re-infection with tuberculosis in areas with a high prevalence, e.g. Africa). As the CD_4 T-lymphocyte count falls there is initially an increase in the

PULMONARY COMPLICATIONS

Infectious diseases
Bacterial infections
  Streptococcus pneumoniae
  Haemophilus influenzae
  Pseudomonas aeruginosa
Tuberculosis
Opportunistic infections
  Fungal
    Pneumocystis carinii
    Aspergillus fumigatus
    Candida albicans
  Viral
    Cytomegalovirus
    Herpes simplex
  Mycobacterial
    Mycobacterium avium-intracellulare

Non-infectious diseases
Neoplastic
  Kaposi's sarcoma
  B-cell lymphoma
Inflammatory
  Lymphocytic alveolitis ($\downarrow T_L\text{co}$)
  Non-specific interstitial pneumonitis
  Lymphocytic interstitial pneumonitis
  Atopic disease (asthma)
  Primary pulmonary hypertension

Infection of the lungs by the HIV virus itself causes a lymphocytic alveolitis with a reduction in the transfer factor for carbon monoxide ($T_L\text{co}$). As the CD_4 T-lymphocyte count falls below 500/μl (normal 600–1600/μl), there is an increased frequency of bacterial infections and tuberculosis. Opportunistic infections (i.e. infections which do not cause disease in immunocompetent individuals) develop as the CD_4 count falls below 200/μl. In the later stages of AIDS, neoplastic diseases (e.g. Kaposi's sarcoma) occur.

Table 8.2 Pulmonary complications of HIV infection.

frequency of infection with common **standard pathogens** (e.g. *Streptococcus pneumoniae, Mycobacterium tuberculosis*). Then as the CD_4 count falls below about 200/µl infections with **opportunistic pathogens** (e.g. *Pneumocystis carinii*) develop. These are infections which do not usually cause disease in immuno-competent people and the occurrence of such opportunistic infections is part of the criteria for diagnosing AIDS ('AIDS-defining illness'). In the later stages of AIDS **neoplastic diseases** (e.g. Kaposi's sarcoma, B-cell lymphomas) occur.

Bacterial respiratory infections

Patients with HIV have an increased incidence of respiratory tract infections with **sinusitis, bronchitis, bronchiectasis** and **pneumonia** occurring due to standard bacterial pathogens. Infection with *Streptococcus pneumoniae, Haemophilus influenzae* and *Staphylococcus aureus* are common, and may precede the diagnosis of HIV infection or the onset of opportunistic infections. Infection with Gram-negative organisms (e.g. *Pseudomonas aeruginosa*) occurs in more advanced disease. The clinical features may be unusual with a higher frequency of complications such as bacteraemia, abscess formation, cavitation and empyema. Pneumococcal and influenza vaccination may be helpful and sometimes long-term prophylactic antibiotics are used.

Pneumocystis carinii pneumonia

Pneumocystis carinii pneumonia (PCP) remains the most common opportunistic infection in AIDS. It is a fungus which only causes disease in immunocompromised individuals, and in HIV infection it typically occurs at the stage when the CD_4 T-lymphocyte count has fallen to below 200/µl. *Pneumocystis carinii* is ubiquitous and asymptomatic infection is common in normal children. PCP typically presents with cough, dyspnoea, fever, hypoxaemia, reduced transfer factor for carbon monoxide and bilateral perihilar interstitial infiltrates on chest X-ray (Fig. 8.1). These clinical features are not specific to PCP and can be caused by a variety of other infections, and more than one pathogen may be present. The chest X-ray may be normal in early PCP and sometimes the radiological features are unusual showing unilateral consolidation, nodules or upper lobe consolidation, for example. Cavitating lesions may occur and pneumothorax is a recognized complication.

Diagnosis

The diagnosis is usually confirmed by detecting *Pneumocystis carinii* using a monoclonal antibody immunofluorescent technique on specimens obtained by **sputum induction** or by bronchoscopy and **bronchoalveolar lavage**. To induce sputum the patient is given 3% hypertonic saline by nebulization followed by chest physiotherapy. If this test is negative it is usual to proceed to bronchoalveolar lavage whereby a bronchoscope is advanced into a subsegmental bronchus and 60 ml aliquots of warmed sterile saline are instilled and aspirated. More invasive procedures, such as **transbronchial** or **surgical lung biopsy**, are usually only performed in complex cases where the aetiology of lung infiltrates cannot be determined by other tests and where a histological diagnosis is considered essential for guiding treatment decisions.

Treatment

Treatment of PCP consists of high-dose intravenous **co-trimoxazole** (trimethoprim 20 mg/kg/day and sulphamethoxazole 100 mg/kg/day in four divided doses) subsequently converted to oral therapy, usually continued for 3 weeks. Side-effects (e.g. allergic rashes, nausea, marrow suppression) are common and intravenous **pentamidine** is an alternative treatment. Patients with moderate or severe PCP (e.g. $Po_2 < 9.5$ kPa (70 mmHg)) benefit from the addition of **corticosteroids** (e.g. prednisolone 40 mg/day) to reduce the pulmonary inflammatory response. High-flow **oxygen** is often required and use of **continuous positive airway pressure (CPAP)** may reduce the need for **ventilation** in severe cases.

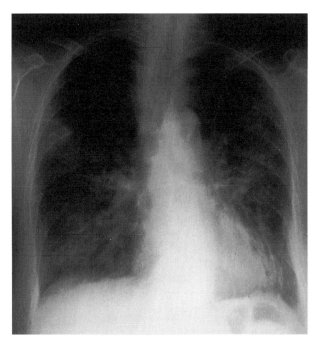

Fig. 8.1 *Pneumocystis carinii* pneumonia. This 28-year-old woman, who was an intravenous drug misuser, presented with fever, dyspnoea and hypoxaemia (Po_2 8.2 kPa (62 mmHg)). Chest X-ray shows diffuse bilateral perihilar and lower zone shadowing. Human immunodeficiency virus (HIV) antibody test was positive and CD_4 T-lymphocyte count was 100/μl (normal 600–1600/μl). Induced sputum was positive for *Pneumocystis carinii* on immunofluorescent monoclonal antibody testing. The patient responded fully to high-dose intravenous co-trimoxazole, prednisolone and oxygen, and she was then commenced on long-term secondary prophylaxis with oral co-trimoxazole 3 days per week.

Prophylaxis

Primary prophylaxis is given to HIV-infected patients whose CD_4 T-cell count is < 200/μl, to prevent first infection. **Secondary prophylaxis** is given to prevent recurrence in patients who have already suffered an episode of PCP. Co-trimoxazole 960 mg given on 3 days per week is the regimen of choice. Nebulized pentamidine given once monthly, or a combination of oral pyrimethamine and dapsone are alternatives for patients who cannot tolerate co-trimoxazole.

Mycobacterial infection

Mycobacterium tuberculosis (see also Chapter 7)

Patients with HIV infection and impaired CD_4 lymphocyte function are highly susceptible to developing **reactivation** of previously acquired latent tuberculosis and to **contracting the disease from an exogenous source**, with rapid **progression to active disease**. In the UK, overlap between the population with HIV infection (mainly young white men) and the population with tuberculosis (mainly older white people and immigrants from the Indian subcontinent) is low so that only about 5% of patients with HIV infection have tuberculosis. However, worldwide it is estimated that **4.5 million people are co-infected with HIV and tuberculosis**, posing a major problem for the global control of tuberculosis. Early in HIV disease, tuberculosis resembles the typical disease seen in non-

HIV patients, with upper lobe consolidation and cavitation. In severely immunocompromised patients the clinical features may be very non-specific with fever, weight loss, malaise, diffuse shadowing on chest X-ray and a high incidence of extrapulmonary disseminated disease. Standard anti-tuberculous treatment is given using isoniazid, rifampicin and pyrazinamide (see Chapter 7) but life-long secondary prophylaxis with isoniazid is recommended. Bacillus Calmette–Guérin (BCG) vaccination is contra-indicated in HIV infection because of the risk of active infection developing with the live attenuated vaccine bacillus in severely immunocompromised patients. Because of their impaired cellular immunity patients with HIV are very susceptible to contracting and transmitting tuberculosis so that strict isolation precautions are warranted, particularly for patients with multi-drug-resistant tuberculosis.

Mycobacterium avium-intracellulare complex

This is an opportunistic mycobacterium which does not usually cause disease in normal subjects but which commonly infects patients with advanced AIDS, particularly when the CD_4 count is < 100/μl. Extrapulmonary disease is more common than pulmonary disease and the diagnosis of disseminated *Mycobacterium avium-intracellulare* complex (MAIC) is usually made when the organism is cultured from blood, bone marrow, lymph node or liver biopsy. The organism is not usually responsive to standard anti-tuberculous drugs and it is treated with a combination of rifabutin, ethambutol, clarithromycin or azithromycin.

Viral infections

Cytomegalovirus (CMV) infection is common in AIDS usually causing systemic infection with hepatitis, retinitis, encephalitis and colitis, rather than overt pulmonary infection. CMV is often isolated from the lungs of AIDS patients but it is not always pathogenic, sometimes being present as a commensal. It is

treated with ganciclovir. **Epstein–Barr virus, adenovirus, influenza** and **herpes simplex virus** may cause pneumonia in AIDS patients. Herpes simplex virus is frequently present in the mouth of HIV-infected patients so that its isolation from the respiratory tract often indicates colonization rather than infection.

Fungal pulmonary infections

Invasive pulmonary infections with *Aspergillus fumigatus* or *Candida albicans* are unusual but may occur late in the course of AIDS. **Cryptococcal** pneumonia may occur as part of a disseminated infection but usually meningoencephalitis dominates the clinical picture. Treatment is with fluconazole or amphotericin. Pulmonary **histoplasmosis** and **coccidioidomycosis** may occur in areas where these fungi are endemic (e.g. USA).

Human immunodeficiency virus-related neoplasms

Kaposi's sarcoma

This is the commonest malignancy in HIV-infected patients. Characteristically it occurs in HIV-infected homosexual men and it is thought that this may relate to co-infection with human herpes virus 8. Pulmonary Kaposi's sarcoma is nearly always accompanied by lesions in the skin or buccal mucosa. Chest X-ray appearances are variable as the tumour may affect the bronchi, lung parenchyma, pleura, or mediastinal lymph nodes. At bronchoscopy Kaposi's sarcoma appears as red or purple lesions. The diagnosis is usually made on the basis of the visual appearances in the context of mucocutaneous Kaposi's sarcoma since biopsy of the bronchial lesions is often non-diagnostic and may cause haemorrhage. Treatment is with anti-neoplastic chemotherapy (e.g. vincristine and bleomycin).

Lymphoma

Late in the course of AIDS, high-grade B-cell lymphomas arise. The lungs are often involved as part of multi-organ involvement. The response to chemotherapy is often poor.

Interstitial pneumonitis

Patients with HIV infection may develop **non-specific interstitial pneumonitis (NIP)**. This presents as episodes of dyspnoea with pulmonary infiltrates, reduced gas diffusion and hypoxaemia. Bronchoalveolar lavage is negative for infection and transbronchial biopsy shows evidence of lymphocytic inflammation. It may be a manifestation of direct HIV infection of the lung. It is often self-limiting but prednisolone may be beneficial.

Lymphoid interstitial pneumonitis is usually seen only in children with HIV infection, and the pneumonitis may be part of more widespread lymphocytic infiltration of liver, bone marrow and parotid glands with hyper-gammaglobulinaemia. Its aetiology is uncertain but it may be related to Epstein–Barr virus co-infection.

Primary pulmonary hypertension

(see Chapter 16)

This is a rare complication of HIV infection and may result from the effect of inflammatory mediators and cytokines, produced by infection of the lung with the HIV virus, on the pulmonary circulation.

Our understanding of HIV infection is progressing very rapidly and anti-retroviral treatments offer great hope for the future. The spectrum of complications of HIV infection is

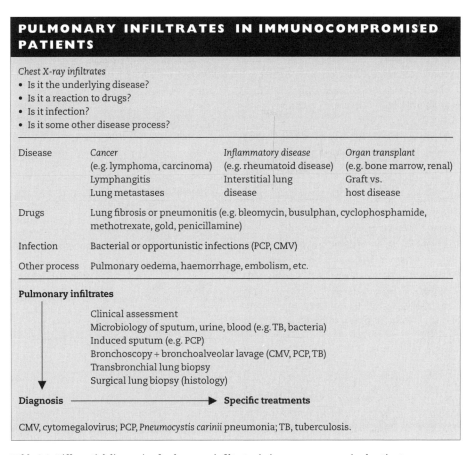

PULMONARY INFILTRATES IN IMMUNOCOMPROMISED PATIENTS

Chest X-ray infiltrates
- Is it the underlying disease?
- Is it a reaction to drugs?
- Is it infection?
- Is it some other disease process?

Disease	Cancer (e.g. lymphoma, carcinoma) Lymphangitis Lung metastases	Inflammatory disease (e.g. rheumatoid disease) Interstitial lung disease	Organ transplant (e.g. bone marrow, renal) Graft vs. host disease
Drugs	Lung fibrosis or pneumonitis (e.g. bleomycin, busulphan, cyclophosphamide, methotrexate, gold, penicillamine)		
Infection	Bacterial or opportunistic infections (PCP, CMV)		
Other process	Pulmonary oedema, haemorrhage, embolism, etc.		

Pulmonary infiltrates

Clinical assessment
Microbiology of sputum, urine, blood (e.g. TB, bacteria)
Induced sputum (e.g. PCP)
Bronchoscopy + bronchoalveolar lavage (CMV, PCP, TB)
Transbronchial lung biopsy
Surgical lung biopsy (histology)

Diagnosis ⟶ **Specific treatments**

CMV, cytomegalovirus; PCP, *Pneumocystis carinii* pneumonia; TB, tuberculosis.

Table 8.3 Differential diagnosis of pulmonary infiltrates in immunocompromised patients.

broad and treatment strategies are complex, requiring specialist knowledge and experience. Preventative strategies (e.g. 'safe sex' practices, needle exchange programmes for drug users) are essential to interrupt the spread of infection.

Other immunocompromised patients

There is an increasing number of patients who are severely immunocompromised by a variety of diseases and by use of immunosuppressive drugs. Patients with neutropenia are particularly vulnerable to **bacterial infections** (e.g. *Streptococcus pneumoniae*, Gram-negative bacteria) and invasive **fungal infections** (e.g. *Aspergillus fumigatus*, *Candida albicans*), and patients with depressed T-lymphocyte function are vulnerable to **PCP**, **tuberculosis** and **cytomegalovirus infection**, for example.

There are three particular situations where profound immunosuppression commonly arises.

1 Patients with cancer receiving **antineoplastic chemotherapy**.

2 Patients with inflammatory diseases (e.g. connective tissue diseases, Wegener's granulomatosis, etc.) receiving **immunosuppressive drugs** (e.g. corticosteroids, cyclophosphamide, methotrexate).

3 Patients post-organ transplantation (bone marrow, renal, lung, etc.) receiving immunosuppressive drugs (e.g. cyclosporin, azathioprine).

The problem is often that of a patient with one of these conditions presenting with pulmonary infiltrates on chest X-ray accompanied by dyspnoea and sometimes fever. The infiltrates in these circumstances may be due to pulmonary involvement by the underlying disease process, a reaction to drug treatment, infection resulting from immunosuppression, or to other coincidental disease processes. Treatment is crucially dependent upon accurate diagnosis.

Assessment involves a careful clinical history and examination focusing on the clinical context and clues to aetiology (Table 8.3). Microbiology of sputum, urine and blood may identify specific pathogens. Induced sputum is particularly useful in diagnosing PCP. If these initial tests are not diagnostic it is often advisable to proceed directly to bronchoscopy with bronchoalveolar lavage for detailed microbiology. Transbronchial lung biopsy is useful in obtaining tissue for histological diagnosis but carries the risk of pneumothorax or haemorrhage. Occasionally surgical lung biopsy is warranted.

Further reading

Cohn JA. Recent advances in HIV infection. *BMJ* 1997; **314**: 487–91.

Delta Coordinating Committee. Delta: a randomized double-blind controlled trial comparing combinations of zidovudine plus didanosine or zalcitabine with zidovudine alone in HIV-infected individuals. *Lancet* 1996; **348**: 283–90.

Lipsky JJ. Antiretroviral drugs for AIDS. *Lancet* 1996; **348**: 800–3.

Miller R. HIV-associated respiratory diseases. *Lancet* 1996; **348**: 307–12.

Quinn TC. Global burden of the HIV pandemic. *Lancet* 1996; **348**: 99–106.

CHAPTER 9

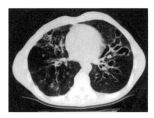

Bronchiectasis and Lung Abscess

Bronchiectasis

Bronchiectasis is a chronic disease characterized by irreversible **dilatation of bronchi** due to bronchial wall damage resulting from infection and inflammation. These morphological changes are usually accompanied by chronic **suppurative lung disease** with cough productive of purulent sputum.

Pathogenesis

Bronchiectasis represents a particular type of bronchial injury which may result from a number of different underlying disease processes. It may be confined to one area of the lung if there is a **local** cause (e.g. bronchial obstruction by a foreign body) or may be **diffuse** if there is a generalized cause (e.g. immunoglobulin deficiency). The walls of the bronchi are infiltrated by inflammatory cells, and are thin and dilated with reduced elastin content. The exact mechanisms giving rise to bronchiectasis are not fully understood but the disease seems to evolve through a vicious circle of steps which may be initiated in a variety of ways (Fig. 9.1):

• **impaired mucociliary clearance** leads to accumulation of secretions;
• accumulated secretions predispose to bacterial **infection**;
• infection provokes an **inflammatory response**, increased mucus production and impaired ciliary function;

• excessive inflammation causes **tissue damage**;
• damage to the bronchial wall produces **dilatation of bronchi** and disruption of mucociliary clearance, and the vicious circle of injury progresses.

Aetiology (Table 9.1)
Infections
Severe infections are one of the commonest causes of bronchial wall damage and bronchiectasis. In childhood, **pertussis** or **measles** are important causes which are declining in frequency due to childhood vaccination programmes. In adults, bronchiectasis may complicate **pneumonia** resulting from virulent organisms such as *Streptococcus pneumoniae*, *Staphylococcus aureus* or *Klebsiella pneumoniae*. Better use of antibiotics has resulted in an overall decline in post-infective bronchiectasis. **Tuberculosis** is still a common cause of bronchiectasis in developing countries. Many adults with **idiopathic** lower lobe bronchiectasis attribute their disease to childhood lung infections, although it is difficult to be sure that such infections played a causative role.

Bronchial obstruction
Bronchiectasis may develop in an area of lung obstructed by a bronchial **carcinoma**. In children, inhalation of a **foreign body** (e.g. peanut) may give rise to bronchial obstruction and distal bronchiectasis. **Lymph node**

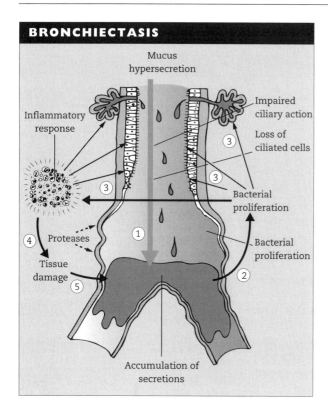

BRONCHIECTASIS

Mucus hypersecretion

Inflammatory response

Impaired ciliary action

Loss of ciliated cells

Bacterial proliferation

Bacterial proliferation

Proteases

Tissue damage

Accumulation of secretions

Fig. 9.1 Bronchiectasis evolves through a vicious circle of steps.

enlargement as part of tuberculosis may compress a bronchus and give rise to bronchiectasis. This particularly occurs in the middle lobe.

Immunodeficiency states

Patients with congenital **hypogammaglobulinaemia** or **selective immunoglobulin deficiencies** usually present with recurrent respiratory tract infections in childhood. Sometimes the diagnosis is not established until adulthood when bronchiectasis may have developed. Serum immunoglobulin levels should be measured in all patients with bronchiectasis since patients with immunoglobulin deficiencies require intravenous immunoglobulin replacement therapy. Immunoglobulin deficiencies may also arise later in life secondary to malignancies such as **lymphoma** or **myeloma**. Patients with **human immunodeficiency virus (HIV) infection** are also

susceptible to recurrent bacterial infections and bronchiectasis (see Chapter 8).

Allergic bronchopulmonary aspergillosis (Fig. 9.2)

Aspergillus fumigatus is a ubiquitous fungus which may **colonize** the respiratory tract as an incidental finding without giving rise to symptoms. Patients with lung cavities (e.g. post-tuberculosis or sarcoidosis) may develop an **aspergilloma**, which is a ball of fungal hyphae which appears on X-ray as a mass in the centre of a cavity surrounded by a halo of radiolucency. This is often asymptomatic, but associated inflammation may cause bronchial artery hypertrophy and haemoptysis requiring surgical resection or therapeutic bronchial artery embolization. **Invasive aspergillosis** (e.g. necrotizing pneumonia or fungaemia) occurs in immunocompromised patients (see Chapter 8).

AETIOLOGY OF BRONCHIECTASIS

Severe infection
  Childhood pertussis
  Bacterial pneumonia
  Recurrent aspiration pneumonia
  Tuberculosis
Bronchial obstruction
  Foreign body (e.g. peanut)
  Bronchial carcinoma
  Lymph node enlargement
Immunodeficient states
  Hypogammaglobulinaemia
  Immunodeficiency due to lymphoma
  HIV infection
Allergic bronchopulmonary aspergillosis
Cystic fibrosis (see Chapter 10)
Ciliary dysfunction
  Primary ciliary dyskinesia
  Kartagener's syndrome
Associated diseases
  Ulcerative colitis
  Rheumatoid arthritis
Idiopathy

Table 9.1 Aetiology of bronchiectasis.

Patients with **asthma** may develop an allergic reaction to *Aspergillus* and demonstrate **precipitating antibodies** to *Aspergillus* in their serum and positive responses to **skin prick tests**. Some of these patients develop **allergic bronchopulmonary aspergillosis** in which there is intense bronchial inflammation with **eosinophilia** and **high IgE** levels in the blood. Eosinophilic infiltrates in the lung give rise to **fleeting X-ray shadows**. Thick **mucus plugs** cause obstruction of small bronchi and give rise to **bronchiectasis** which is usually proximal in location. Treatment requires suppression of the inflammatory immune response by oral prednisolone and high-dose inhaled steroids.

Ciliary dyskinesia

The epithelial cells of the bronchi possess cilia which beat in an organized way so as to move particles in the layer of mucus on their surface upwards and out of the lung. This **mucociliary** escalator is an essential clearance mechanism. Ciliary function is impaired by cigarette smoke and bacterial toxins. Viral infections may cause widespread shedding of ciliated respiratory cells. Bronchial damage of whatever cause often disrupts the mucociliary clearance mechanism impairing the lung defence mechanisms and perpetuating the vicious circle of bronchiectasis.

  Primary ciliary dyskinesia is an autosomal recessive condition in which there is an abnormality of the ultrastructure of cilia throughout the body such that they do not beat in a coordinated fashion. Failure of ciliary function in the respiratory tract gives rise to sinusitis and bronchiectasis. The tail of sperm is also a cilial structure and males with primary ciliary dyskinesia are infertile. It is thought that cilia are also responsible for the normal rotation of internal structures in embryonic life so that failure of ciliary function results in random rotation with about 50% of patients having dextrocardia and situs inversus (e.g. appendix in left iliac fossa). Ciliary dyskinesia with situs inversus. is known as **Kartagener's syndrome**.

  Mucociliary clearance can be assessed by measuring the rate of removal from the lung of an inhaled radiolabelled aerosol. The ultrastructure of cilia can be studied by electron microscopy. Ciliary function can also be studied by microscope photometry which assesses the beat frequency of cilia obtained by brush biopsy of nasal mucosa. A bedside estimate of ciliary function can be obtained by timing the nasal clearance of saccharin. In this test a 1 mm cube of saccharin is placed on the inferior turbinate of the nose. The time from placing the particle to the patient tasting the saccharin is usually less than 30 minutes, and is a measure of nasal ciliary clearance. In men, sperm motility may be assessed by microscopy of seminal fluid.

Associated diseases

Patients with certain diseases seem to have an increased incidence of bronchiectasis. These diseases include rheumatoid arthritis, ulcera-

ASPERGILLUS LUNG DISEASE

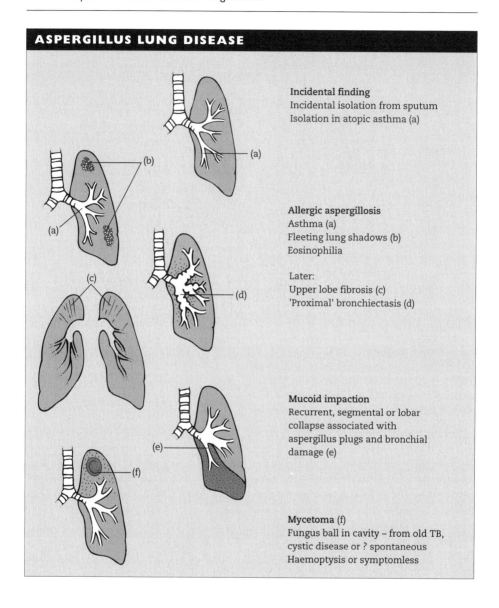

Incidental finding
Incidental isolation from sputum
Isolation in atopic asthma (a)

Allergic aspergillosis
Asthma (a)
Fleeting lung shadows (b)
Eosinophilia

Later:
Upper lobe fibrosis (c)
'Proximal' bronchiectasis (d)

Mucoid impaction
Recurrent, segmental or lobar
collapse associated with
aspergillus plugs and bronchial
damage (e)

Mycetoma (f)
Fungus ball in cavity – from old TB,
cystic disease or ? spontaneous
Haemoptysis or symptomless

Fig. 9.2 Summary of the clinical spectrum of *Aspergillus* lung disease.

tive colitis, Crohn's disease and coeliac disease but the mechanism by which bronchiectasis arises in these diseases is unclear.

Clinical features

The cardinal feature of bronchiectasis is **chronic cough** productive of copious **purulent sputum**. There is considerable variation in the severity of the disease and mild cases are often misdiagnosed as chronic bronchitis. **Haemoptysis** is common and may occasionally be severe requiring therapeutic embolization of hypertrophied bronchial arteries to control the bleeding source. Infective exacerbations may be associated with **fever** and **pleuritic pain**. Chronic severe bronchiectasis

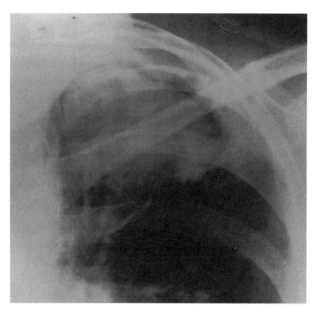

Fig. 9.3 This 70-year-old woman had suffered from tuberculosis in the 1950s which had resulted in bilateral apical lung fibrosis and severely impaired lung function (forced expiratory volume in 1 second, 0.5 litre; forced vital capacity, 1.1 litre). She presented with recurrent major haemoptysis, and chest X-ray showed features characteristic of an aspergilloma with an opacity in the left apex surrounded by a halo of radiolucency. *Aspergillus* hyphae were seen on sputum microscopy and *Aspergillus* precipitins were present in her blood. Tests for carcinoma and tuberculosis were negative. Bronchial arteriography showed marked hypertrophy of the bronchial artery to the left upper lobe and therapeutic embolization was performed resulting in resolution of the haemoptysis.

may cause **malaise**, **weight loss** and **halitosis** (foul breath). Coarse **crackles** may be audible over affected areas and **clubbing** is common. Systemic spread of infection (e.g. cerebral abscess) and secondary amyloidosis are now very rare because of control of infection by antibiotics.

Investigations

A **chest X-ray** may show features of bronchiectasis such as peribronchial thickening, which is evident as parallel tramline shadowing, or cystic dilated bronchi. However, the chest X-ray is often normal in less severe cases and high-resolution **computed tomography (CT)** is the key investigation in confirming the diagnosis and in determining the location and extent of the disease. Bronchography, in which the bronchial tree is outlined by instillation of a radiocontrast dye, has been superseded by CT scanning (Fig. 9.4).

Having confirmed the presence of bronchiectasis, an attempt should be made to diagnose the underlying cause of the bronchiectasis, and further specific tests performed as indicated, e.g. ***Aspergillus*** **precipitins** and skin prick tests (allergic bronchopulmonary aspergillosis), **immunoglobulin levels** and IgG subclasses (hypogammaglobulinaemia), **sweat tests** (cystic fibrosis), **and ciliary function tests** (ciliary dyskinesia). **Bronchoscopy** is useful in detecting any endobronchial obstruction in cases of localized bronchiectasis. **Sputum microbiology** should be performed to define what infective organisms are present as a guide to antibiotic treatment. **Lung function tests** define the level of any deficit and help determine whether bronchodilator drugs may be helpful.

Treatment

• **Specific treatment** of the underlying cause is rarely possible but relief of endo-bronchial obstruction (e.g. foreign body) is the key treatment for some patients, intravenous immunoglobulin replacement therapy is essential for patients with hypogammaglobulinaemia, and suppression of the inflammatory response by oral or inhaled corticosteroids is important in allergic aspergillosis.

• **Chest physiotherapy** is the most effective treatment in preventing the accumulation of secretions. Postural drainage (using gravity-assisted positions to aid clearance of secretions from affected areas), percussion and forced expiratory techniques ('huffing') should be guided by a physiotherapist.

• **Antibiotics** are used to suppress chronic infection and to treat exacerbations. High doses are required to penetrate the scarred bronchial mucosa and purulent secretions. The choice of antibiotics is guided by the results of sputum microbiology. *Haemophilus influenzae* and *Streptococcus pneumoniae* are common and are usually sensitive to amoxycillin. Antibiotic resistance may develop, and the presence of co-infection with *Moraxella catarrhalis* is usually associated with the production of β-lactamase so that co-amoxyclav or ciprofloxacin may be useful. *Pseudomonas aeruginosa* is common in severe disease and may be treated by oral ciprofloxacin or intravenous anti-pseudomonal antibiotics (e.g. azlocillin, ceftazidime, gentamicin). Nebulized antibiotics (e.g. colistin) may be used to suppress chronic *Pseudomonas* infection. Long-term oral antibiotics (e.g. amoxycillin) are sometimes used in severe disease but there is a risk of promoting antibiotic resistance. Anaerobic infections (e.g. *Bacteroides*) are quite common and respond to metronidazole. Pneumococcal and influenza vaccinations are recommended for patients with bronchiectasis.

• **Bronchodilator drugs** (e.g. salbutamol,

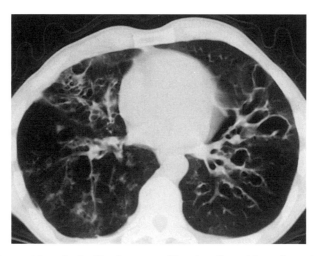

Fig. 9.4 This 50-year-old man had suffered pertussis pneumonia at the age of 18 months. He had chronic cough productive of copious purulent sputum isolating *Pseudomonas aeruginosa* on culture. Computed tomography showed extensive bilateral bronchiectasis with dilatation of bronchi, cyst formation and patchy peribronchial consolidation. He was treated with postural drainage physiotherapy, salbutamol, long-term nebulized antibiotics (colistin) and intermittent courses of oral ciprofloxacin or intravenous ceftazidime and gentamicin.

terbutaline) and an **inhaled steroid** (e.g. beclomethasone, budesonide, fluticasone) are indicated where there is associated reversible airways obstruction.

• **Surgical excision** is a potential treatment for the few patients who have localized disease and troublesome symptoms. **Lung transplantation** is an option for patients whose disease has progressed to respiratory failure.

Lung abscess (Fig. 9.5)

A lung abscess is a **localized collection of pus within a cavitated necrotic lesion in the lung parenchyma**. The chest X-ray characteristically shows a cavitating lesion containing a fluid level. The patient typically complains of cough with expectoration of large amounts of foul material often accompanied by haemoptysis, fever, weight loss and malaise. It is important to distinguish between a lung abscess and other causes of cavitating lung lesions, such as a squamous cell carcinoma, and bronchoscopy or percutaneous fine-needle aspiration of the lesion may be required.

Fig. 9.5 Aetiology of lung abscess.

The infection giving rise to a lung abscess may arise via a number of routes. Oropharyngeal **aspiration** is the commonest cause and occurs in states of unconsciousness (e.g. alcohol excess, epilepsy, anaesthesia), and where there is dysphagia due to oesophageal or neuromuscular disease. Infection of the upper airways (e.g. sinusitis, dental abscess) may be an important source of bacteria, and anaerobic organism (e.g. *Bacteroides*, *Streptococcus milleri*) are common. Infection may arise distal to **bronchial obstruction** caused by a tumour or foreign body (e.g. inhaled peanut). The centre of an area of destructive **pneumonia** may break down to form a lung abscess particularly when the pneumonia is due to *Staphylococcus aureus* or *Klebsiella pneumoniae*. Tuberculosis may present as a lung abscess. **Blood-borne** infection may occur by intravenous injection of infected material by drug addicts. Pulmonary emboli may cause pulmonary infarction, with secondary infection giving rise to an abscess. Penetrating **chest trauma** is an unusual cause of lung abscess. **Transdiaphragmatic** spread of infection may occur from a subphrenic abscess (e.g. postcholecystectomy) or a hepatic abscess (e.g. amoebic abscess).

Drainage of pus from the abscess cavity is a

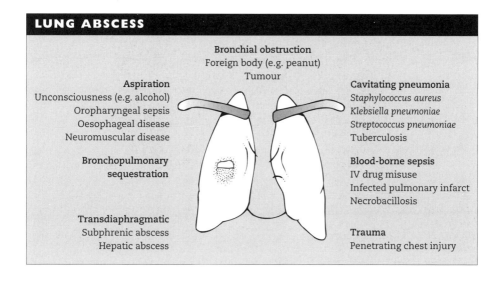

LUNG ABSCESS

Bronchial obstruction
Foreign body (e.g. peanut)
Tumour

Aspiration
Unconsciousness (e.g. alcohol)
Oropharyngeal sepsis
Oesophageal disease
Neuromuscular disease

Bronchopulmonary
sequestration

Transdiaphragmatic
Subphrenic abscess
Hepatic abscess

Cavitating pneumonia
Staphylococcus aureus
Klebsiella pneumoniae
Streptococcus pneumoniae
Tuberculosis

Blood-borne sepsis
IV drug misuse
Infected pulmonary infarct
Necrobacillosis

Trauma
Penetrating chest injury

key aspect of treatment. This can often be achieved by bronchial drainage using postural drainage physiotherapy. Sometimes percutaneous drainage is achieved by positioning a catheter drainage tube under radiological guidance. Prolonged **antibiotic** therapy is given in accordance with the likely organism and the results of microbiology tests (e.g. metronidazole for anaerobic infections). **Surgical excision** of the abscess cavity is sometimes required where medical treatment fails.

Necrobacillosis

Necrobacillosis (Lemière's disease) is an unusual cause of lung abscess which is associated with a very characteristic clinical picture first described by Lemière. Typically a young adult develops a **severe sore throat** with **cervical adenopathy** due to infection with the anaerobe, *Fusobacterium necrophorum*. This is associated with a local venulitis followed by a **septicaemic illness** with haematogenous spread of infection. The lungs are frequently involved with multiple **abscesses** forming, often with a **pleural empyema** and evidence of infection elsewhere, e.g. **septic arthritis**, **osteomyelitis**. Prolonged anaerobic blood culture is required to identify the organism, which is sensitive to metronidazole.

Bronchopulmonary sequestration

Bronchopulmonary sequestration is a congenital anomaly in which an **area of lung is not connected to the bronchial tree** (i.e. 'sequestered') and has an **anomalous blood supply** usually from the aorta. If infection develops in the sequestration it often progresses to an abscess because of lack of drainage to the bronchial tree. Surgical resection is required but pre-operative bronchial arteriography is necessary to identify the anomalous blood supply.

Further reading

Chapel HM. Consensus on diagnosis and management of primary antibody deficiencies. *BMJ* 1994; **308**: 581–5.

Chippindale AJ, Patel B, Mamtora H. A case of necrobacillosis. *Thorax* 1990; **45**: 74–5.

Ellis DA, Thornley PE, Wightman AJ *et al.* Present outlook in bronchiectasis: clinical and social study and review of factors influencing prognosis. *Thorax* 1981; **36**: 659–64.

Munro NC, Cooke JC, Currie DC *et al.* Comparison of thin section computed tomography with bronchography for identifying bronchiectatic segments in patients with chronic sputum production. *Thorax* 1990; **45**: 135–9.

Neild JE, Eykyn SJ, Phillips I. Lung abscess and empyema. *Q J Med* 1985; **57**: 875–82.

CHAPTER 10

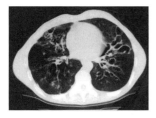

Cystic Fibrosis

Introduction

Cystic fibrosis is the commonest potentially lethal inherited disease of Caucasians. **It affects about 1 in 2500 live births** in the UK and is inherited in an autosomal recessive manner. About **1 in 25 of the population is a carrier** of the disease.

The basic defect

Cystic fibrosis is due to a defect in a gene on the long arm of chromosome 7 which codes for a 1480-amino-acid protein, named **cystic fibrosis transmembrane conductance regulator (CFTR)**. More than 400 mutations of this gene have been identified but the commonest is designated ΔF508, in which mutation of a single codon of the gene results in the loss of phenylalanine ('delta F') at position 508 of the protein. CFTR functions as a **chloride channel** in the membrane of epithelial cells and the primary physiological defect in cystic fibrosis is reduced chloride conductance at epithelial membranes, most notably in the respiratory, gastrointestinal, pancreatic, hepato-biliary and reproductive tracts. In sweat ducts, failure to reabsorb chloride ions results in elevated concentrations of chloride and sodium in the sweat, a characteristic feature of the disease and the basis for the sweat test used in diagnosis.

Lungs

In the bronchial mucosa failure of chloride transport results in **secretions of abnormal viscosity** which interfere with mucociliary clearance and permit the adherence of bacteria to the mucosa. The inflammatory response is unable to clear the infection and a vicious cycle of **infection** and **inflammation** develops, progressing to lung damage, **bronchiectasis**, **respiratory failure** and **death**.

Gastrointestinal tract

In the **pancreas** the abnormal ion transport results in the plugging and obstruction of ductules with progressive destruction of the gland. The pancreatic enzymes (e.g. lipase) fail to reach the small intestine and this results in **malabsorption** of fats with steatorrhoea and failure to gain weight. Progressive destruction of the endocrine pancreas may cause **diabetes**. Abnormalities of bile secretion and absorption cause an increased incidence of **gallstones** and **biliary cirrhosis**. Sludging and desiccation of intestinal contents probably accounts for the occurrence of **meconium ileus** (neonatal intestinal obstruction) in about 10% of babies with cystic fibrosis, and for the development of **distal intestinal obstruction syndrome** (meconium ileus equivalent) in older children and adults.

CYSTIC FIBROSIS

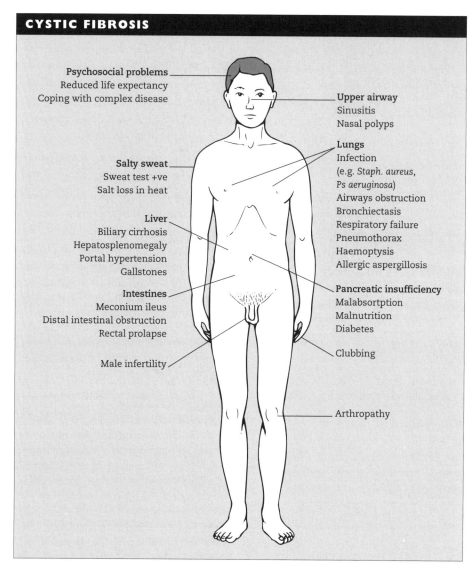

Psychosocial problems
Reduced life expectancy
Coping with complex disease

Upper airway
Sinusitis
Nasal polyps

Lungs
Infection
(e.g. *Staph. aureus*,
Ps aeruginosa)
Airways obstruction
Bronchiectasis
Respiratory failure
Pneumothorax
Haemoptysis
Allergic aspergillosis

Salty sweat
Sweat test +ve
Salt loss in heat

Liver
Biliary cirrhosis
Hepatosplenomegaly
Portal hypertension
Gallstones

Intestines
Meconium ileus
Distal intestinal obstruction
Rectal prolapse

Pancreatic insufficiency
Malabsortption
Malnutrition
Diabetes

Clubbing

Male infertility

Arthropathy

Fig. 10.1 Clinical features of cystic fibrosis. Cystic fibrosis is a multi-system disease resulting from mutations of the gene which codes for a protein, cystic fibrosis transmembrane conductance regulator (CTFR), which functions as a chloride channel on epithelial membranes. Failure of chloride conductance results in abnormal secretions and organ damage in the respiratory, pancreatic, hepatobiliary, gastrointestinal and reproductive tracts.

Clinical features (Fig. 10.1)

Infants and young children

About 10% of children with cystic fibrosis present at birth with **meconium ileus**, a form of intestinal obstruction caused by inspissated viscid faecal material resulting from lack of pancreatic enzymes and from reduced intestinal water secretion. More than half of children affected by cystic fibrosis have obvious malabsorption by the age of 6 months with **failure**

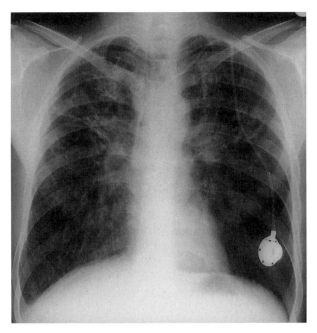

Fig. 10.2 Chest X-ray of this 37-year-old man with cystic fibrosis shows hyperinflation, peribronchial thickening, cystic bronchiectasis and perihilar fibrosis. A Portacath central venous system is in place with the access port situated subcutaneously in the left lower chest. He has chronic *Pseudomonas aeruginosa* infection and receives about three courses of intravenous ceftazidime and gentamicin at home each year. His forced expiratory volume in 1 second is 1.5 litres (42% of predicted) and his general condition and lung function have remained stable over the last 5 years on treatment including long-term nebulized colistin, nebulized deoxyribonuclease, physiotherapy and nutritional supplements.

to thrive associated with abdominal distension and copious offensive stools from **steatorrhoea** due to malabsorbed fat. **Rectal prolapse** occasionally occurs. Recurrent **respiratory infections** rapidly become a prominent feature with cough, sputum production and wheeze.

Older children and adults
Respiratory disease (Fig. 10.2)
Persistent cough and purulent sputum characterize the development of **bronchiectasis**. Progressive lung damage is associated with the development of digital clubbing and progressive **airways obstruction**, sometimes associated with wheeze. Serial measurements of forced expiratory volume in 1 second (FEV_1) give an indication of the severity and progression of the disease. Some patients show a significant asthmatic component with reversible airways obstruction and some develop colonization of the bronchi by *Aspergillus fumigatus* and may show features of allergic bronchopulmonary aspergillosis (see Chapter 9). Initially the typical organisms isolated on sputum cultures are **Staphylococcus aureus**, *Haemophilus influenzae* and *Streptococcus pneumoniae*. By teenage years many have become infected with mucoid strains of **Pseudomonas aeruginosa**. **Burkholderia cepacia** is a Gramnegative organism that causes onion rot and is not usually pathogenic in humans, but it may infect patients with cystic fibrosis and can be transmitted from one patient to another by close contact. The clinical course of patients with *Burkholderia cepacia* infection is very variable but some show a rapid decline in lung function after contracting infection.

As the cycle of infection and inflammation progresses, lung damage worsens with deteriorating airways obstruction, destruction of lung parenchyma, impairment of gas exchange and the development of **hypoxaemia**, **hypercapnia** and **cor pulmonale**. The persistent pulmonary inflammation provokes hypertrophy of the bronchial arteries, and **haemoptysis** becomes common. Occasionally when severe bleeding occurs therapeutic embolization of the bronchial arteries may be required. **Pneumothorax** occurs in about 5–10% of patients with advanced disease and may require prompt tube drainage. Pleurodesis may be required for recurrent pneumothoraces but this should be performed with care so as not to compromise future potential lung transplantation.

Gastrointestinal disease

About 85% of patients with cystic fibrosis have **pancreatic insufficiency** with **malabsorption of fat** due to lack of lipase. Unless these patients receive adequate pancreatic enzyme supplements they develop steatorrhoea with frequent bulky offensive stools and failure to gain weight. Progressive destruction of the endocrine pancreas is manifest by an increasing incidence of **diabetes** as these patients get older. A variety of **hepatobiliary abnormalities** occur including fatty liver, gallstones and focal biliary fibrosis, and about 5% of patients develop multi-nodular cirrhosis with hepatosplenomegaly, portal hypertension, oesophageal varices and liver failure. **Distal intestinal obstruction syndrome** (meconium ileus equivalent) (Fig. 10.3) results from inspissated, fatty, semi-solid faecal material obstructing the terminal ileum. A number of factors contribute to the development of this complication including malabsorption of fat, disordered intestinal motility and dehydrated intestinal contents resulting from defective intestinal chloride transport. The clinical features vary depending on the severity of the obstruction. Typically the patient suffers recurrent episodes of colicky abdominal pain and constipation, and there is often a palpable mass in the right iliac fossa. In severe cases complete intestinal obstruction may develop with abdominal distension, vomiting and multiple fluid levels in distended small bowel on an erect X-ray of abdomen. It is treated by administration of the radiocontrast Gastrografin (sodium diatrizoate). This agent has detergent properties which allow it to penetrate the inspissated fatty material and its hypertonicity then draws fluid into the faecal bolus. In the absence of complete obstruction the bowel can be flushed using balanced intestinal lavage solution. Other measures include rehydration, stool softeners (e.g. lactulose) and N-acetylcysteine which probably acts by cleaving disulphide bonds in the mucoprotein faecal bolus. Prevention of recurrence requires adequate pancreatic enzyme supplements, avoidance of dehydration and sometimes use of prokinetic agents such as cisapride.

Other complications

Nearly all **male patients are infertile** due to congenital bilateral absence of the vas deferens. The exact mechanism by which this complication occurs is not known but it has been suggested that it may result from resorption of the vas deferens after it has become plugged with viscid secretions in fetal life. Females have near normal fertility although some abnormalities of cervical mucus are present. **Pregnancy** places additional burdens on the mother's health and is sometimes associated with a deterioration in the disease because of increased nutritional stress and impaired bronchial clearance. However, the main risk is of the mother failing to maintain all aspects of her own treatment as she focuses on the care of the baby.

Upper airway involvement causes troublesome **sinusitis** and **nasal polyps**. Cystic fibrosis **arthropathy** probably results from the deposition in joints of antigen–antibody complexes produced by the immune response to bacterial lung infections. Vasculitic **rashes** may also occur. In hot weather, patients with cystic fibrosis are at risk of developing **heat prostration** due to excess loss of salt in

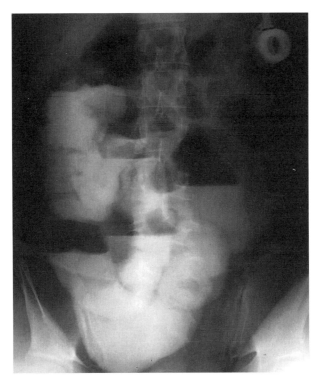

Fig. 10.3 Meconium ileus equivalent. This 31-year-old woman with cystic fibrosis was admitted to hospital complaining of abdominal distension, colicky pain and constipation. A mass of inspissated faecal material was palpable in the right iliac fossa. Erect abdominal X-ray (after taking Gastrografin) shows distended loops of small bowel containing multiple fluid levels. A diagnosis of meconium ileus equivalent (distal intestinal obstruction syndrome) was made and she was treated with Gastrografin (orally and by enema), N-acetylcysteine orally, intravenous fluids, followed by flushing of the bowel using balanced intestinal lavage solution.

sweat. As these patients are living longer, a number of other complications are being described such as **osteoporosis** and **amyloidosis**. Patients with cystic fibrosis face major **social and emotional stresses** relating to their reduced life expectancy, outlook for employment, ability to form relationships and undertake marriage, and their general capacity to cope with a complex disease and its treatment.

Diagnosis

The diagnosis of cystic fibrosis has classically been based upon the demonstration of **el-evated sweat sodium and chloride** concentrations on a sweat test, in association with **characteristic clinical features** such as recurrent respiratory infections and evidence of pancreatic insufficiency. Nowadays the diagnosis is usually confirmed by the demonstration of **two known cystic fibrosis mutations** (e.g. ΔF508|ΔF508) on DNA analysis.

Sweat testing

In cystic fibrosis the ion-transport defect results in a failure to reabsorb chloride ions from the sweat, so that elevated sweat chloride and sodium concentrations are a characteristic feature of the disease. Sweating is induced by

pilocarpine iontophoresis, the sweat is collected on filter paper and then analysed for sodium and chloride. Pilocarpine is placed on the skin of the forearm and a small electrical current is passed across it to enhance its penetration of the skin and stimulation of the sweat ducts. Meticulous technique is required to avoid evaporation of secretions or contamination. At least 100 mg of sweat are required for accurate analysis and sweat sodium and chloride levels above 70 mmol/L on repeated tests are abnormal.

DNA analysis

The discovery of the cystic fibrosis gene in 1989 led to the development of **genotyping as an aid to diagnosis**. Genotyping can also be used to detect **carrier status**, and can be applied to chorionic villus biopsy material for **antenatal diagnosis**. However, there are more than 500 mutations of the cystic fibrosis gene currently identified and it is only possible to test for the more common mutations so that it can be difficult to exclude cystic fibrosis due to rare mutations. DNA analysis has established the diagnosis in some individuals with only mild clinical features, and this has extended our knowledge of the clinical spectrum of the disease to include some very rare older, less severely affected patients. Affected individuals have two gene mutations (e.g. ΔF508|ΔF508), one inherited from each of their parents. Carriers of the disease have only one abnormal gene, and do not show any evidence of the disease.

Screening

Early diagnosis of cystic fibrosis allows specific treatment to be commenced rapidly, and this is associated with an improved prognosis. Infants with cystic fibrosis have elevated serum **immunoreactive trypsin activity**. This can be measured on a single dried blood spot obtained on a Guthrie card as part of the neonatal screening programme for diseases such as phenylketonuria and hypothyroidism.

Treatment (Fig. 10.4)

Cystic fibrosis is a complex multi-system disease, and skills from several disciplines are needed in treating these patients. The optimal use of currently available treatments and the introduction of new treatments is best achieved by concentrating the care of these patients in regional **specialist centres**. The basic elements of treatment comprise clearance of bronchial secretions by **physiotherapy**, treatment of pulmonary infection by **antibiotics** and correction of nutritional deficits by use of **pancreatic enzyme supplements** and **dietary support**. Patients and their families require continuous encouragement and support in coping with this complex disease. The Cystic Fibrosis Trust acts as a focus of **information and support**, and co-ordinates fund raising for research.

Chest physiotherapy

The viscid purulent sputum results in airways obstruction, and clearance of airway secretions by chest physiotherapy is important at all stages of the disease. A variety of techniques can be used including **postural drainage** (using gravity-assisted positions to aid drainage), chest **percussion** and **positive expiratory pressure devices** to aid dislodgement and expectoration of sputum from the peripheral airways. As patients mature it is important that they learn to perform bronchial clearance themselves. The 'active cycle of breathing technique' is often effective and popular with adult patients. This involves a **cycle of breathing control**, thoracic expansion exercises and the **forced expiratory technique** ('huffing') which releases secretions from peripheral bronchi. Exercise is an excellent adjunct to physiotherapy but should not replace it.

Antibiotics

Children with cystic fibrosis should be **immunized** against pertussis and measles as part of the childhood vaccination programme,

PATHOPHYSIOLOGY AND TREATMENT OF CF

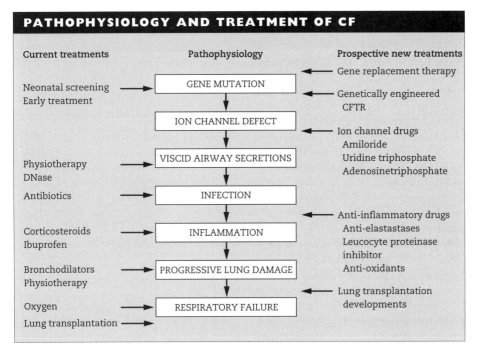

Fig. 10.4 Summary of pathophysiology and treatment of cystic fibrosis lung disease. The genetic defect results in a lack of cystic fibrosis transmembrane conductance regulator (CFTR) and abnormal chloride transport in airway epithelium. The resultant viscid secretions predispose to the acquisition and persistence of bacterial infection. The inflammatory response is unable to clear infection and a vicious cycle of infection and inflammation causes bronchiectasis and progressive lung damage, leading to respiratory failure and death, over a median period of 30 years. Key elements of treatment at all stages of the disease are nutrition, antibiotics, chest physiotherapy and psychosocial support. A variety of currently available and prospective treatments target the different pathophysiological stages of the disease to improve the outlook for patients with cystic fibrosis.

and should receive annual influenza vaccination thereafter. They should avoid contact with people with respiratory infections and avoid inhalation of cigarette smoke. A variety of antibiotic strategies are used. *Staphylococcus aureus* is a major pathogen in the disease from early childhood and long-term continuous **flucloxacillin** is often used to suppress this infection. Further oral antibiotics are given during exacerbations in accordance with sputum cultures and sensitivity testing. Common pathogens include *Haemophilus influenzae* and *Streptococcus pneumoniae* which are usually sensitive to **amoxycillin**.

Infection with *Pseudomonas aeruginosa*
becomes an increasing problem as children get older, and an important strategy in antibiotic therapy is to postpone for as long as possible the colonization of the airways by this organism. Frequent sputum cultures are performed and intensive anti-pseudomonal antibiotic therapy is given when the organism is first isolated. This often comprises an **initial prolonged course of oral ciprofloxacin** and **nebulized colistin**. If this does not eradicate infection then **intravenous anti-pseudomonal antibiotics** are recommended. Eventually chronic infection with *Pseudomonas aeruginosa* becomes established. Attempts at suppressing the effects of this

infection involve long-term use of **nebulized antibiotics** such as colistin or tobramycin with additional courses of intravenous anti-pseudomonal antibiotics during infective exacerbations or when there is a decline in lung function. Usually an aminoglycoside (e.g. gentamicin, amikacin) is given in combination with a third-generation cephalosporin (e.g. ceftazidime) or a modified penicillin (e.g. azlocillin). Treatment is usually given for 14 days and high doses are required to achieve adequate penetration of antibiotics into scarred bronchial mucosa and because patients with cystic fibrosis have increased renal clearance of antibiotics.

Intravenous antibiotic treatment is often given **at home** by the patient after training. Where venous access is difficult a totally implanted central venous device can be inserted (e.g. Portacath). This comprises a central venous cannula connected to a subcutaneous port which is accessed by inserting a special non-cutting needle through the skin and the diaphragm of the subcutaneous chamber.

Burkholderia cepacia is usually resistant to many of the commonly used anti-pseudomonal antibiotics such as colistin, ciprofloxacin and aminoglycosides, but is often sensitive to ceftazidime, imipenem or meropenem. Because of the potential for transmission of *Burkholderia cepacia* between patients with cystic fibrosis, patients with this infection should be **segregated** from other cystic fibrosis patients and should be seen in separate clinics and segregated during hospitalization.

Bronchodilator medication

Some patients with cystic fibrosis have a reversible component to their airways obstruction, and benefit from bronchodilator drugs (e.g. salbutamol, terbutaline) and inhaled steroids (e.g. beclomethasone, budesonide, fluticasone).

Deoxyribonuclease

The sputum of patients with cystic fibrosis contains high levels of DNA which is derived from the nuclei of decaying neutrophils. This makes the sputum very viscid and difficult to expectorate. Recombinant human deoxyribonuclease (DNase) is a genetically engineered enzyme which cleaves DNA. This recently developed treatment can be administered by nebulization and improves the lung function and reduces the number of exacerbations in some patients.

Anti-inflammatory drugs

The inflammatory response is unable to eradicate infection and contributes to the progressive lung damage. Corticosteroid drugs (e.g. **prednisolone**) may have a beneficial effect but their use is limited by side-effects. High-dose **ibuprofen** may also be useful in reducing lung injury by inhibiting the migration and activation of neutrophils.

Nutrition

Pancreatic enzyme supplements (e.g. Creon, Pancrease, Nutrizym) are taken with each meal and with snacks containing fat. Enteric-coated preparations protect the lipase from inactivation by gastric acid, and use of antacid medication (e.g. cimetidine, ranitidine) may improve effectiveness. The dose of enzyme is adjusted according to the dietary intake to optimize weight gain and growth and to control steatorrhoea. Use of high doses of pancreatic enzymes has been associated with the development of strictures of the ascending colon — so-called 'fibrosing colonopathy' — in a small number of children so that it is recommended that the dose of lipase should not exceed 10 000 U/kg/day. Supplements of **fat-soluble vitamins** (A, D, E, K) are routinely given.

Patients with cystic fibrosis suffer from nutritional deficiencies as a result of malabsorption and the increased energy requirements resulting from increased energy expenditure due to chronic lung infection. Most patients with cystic fibrosis require 120–150% of the recommended daily calorie intake for normal individuals, so that healthy eating for a patient with cystic fibrosis includes **high-energy foods** and frequent snacks between main meals. **Dietary supplements** (e.g. Fortisip, Scandishake) are useful when factors such as anorexia limit intake. In advanced disease **nocturnal enteral feeding** of high-energy formulas, through a nasogastric tube or gastrostomy, may be required.

Advanced disease

The clinical course of cystic fibrosis is very variable but an FEV_1 of less then 30% of the predicted value, for example, is associated with a 50% 2-year mortality rate. An awareness of the stage of the disease and the likely prognosis assists in planned management. Oxygen saturation should be measured by oximetry at each clinic visit in patients with advanced disease and when hypoxaemia develops domiciliary **oxygen** may alleviate the complications of respiratory failure. **Lung transplantation** is the main option to be considered for patients with advanced disease but the lack of donor organs severely limits the use of this treatment (see Chapter 20). Many patients will opt for a **palliative care** approach avoiding unpleasant interventions and focusing on measures which alleviate symptoms. Death is usually peaceful after a short coma due to ventilatory failure.

Prognosis (Fig. 10.5)

The prognosis of patients with cystic fibrosis

has improved dramatically over the years. In the 1950s, survival beyond 10 years was unusual. Now the median survival is about 30 years and it is predicted to be at least 40 years for children born in the 1990s. There are now about 6250 patients with cystic fibrosis in the UK, of whom 40% are adults (aged 16 or over). Patients entering adulthood with cystic fibrosis face a number of problems, particularly relating to their chronic lung disease and reduced life expectancy (e.g. life insurance, choice of career, relationships, marriage, pregnancy, fertility). The improved survival of patients with cystic fibrosis has been attributed to a combination of factors including improved management of meconium ileus in neonates, earlier diagnosis, better dietary management and pancreatic enzyme supplementation and meticulous attention to physiotherapy and antibiotic treatments in specialist centres.

Prospective treatments

The identification of the cystic fibrosis gene in 1989 revolutionized our understanding of the detailed pathophysiology of this disease and new treatments are being directed at each stage of the disease process. Perhaps the most exciting approach to treatment is the direct replacement of the defective gene by **gene therapy**.

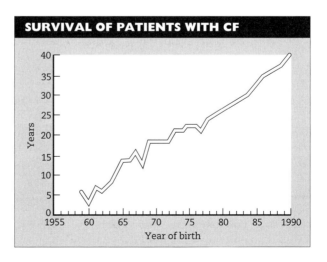

Fig. 10.5 Projected median survival of patients with cystic fibrosis by year of birth from 1959 to 1990. (Reproduced with permission from Elborn et al., 1991.)

The DNA of CFTR has been cloned and has been given to patients in experimental trials using a vector such as a modified adenovirus or liposome to introduce the gene into epithelial cells. Expression of the gene can be detected by measuring transepithelial potential differences. However, many practical difficulties have to be overcome before gene therapy can be considered as a clinically effective treatment for patients. New pharmacological approaches are being attempted to correct the **ion transport** defect by stimulating alternative chloride channels or inhibiting sodium channels. Nebulized amiloride has been shown to have a small effect in that regard, and newer agents such as adenosine triphosphate (ATP) and uridine triphosphate (UTP) are being assessed. **Nebulized DNase** represents a novel approach to reducing the viscosity of the sputum. This drug is currently available and improves the lung function and reduces the number of exacerbations in some patients. Attempts at modifying the inflammatory response involve the assessment of the role of some currently available (e.g. ibuprofen) and some novel **anti-inflammatory agents** (e.g. pentoxifylline, anti-elastases, serum leucocyte proteinase inhibitors (SLPI)). Improvements in the field of **lung transplantation** offer the best hope for patients in the advanced stages of the disease. Advances in many different areas of scientific research are being brought into clinical practice in order to improve the outlook for patients with cystic fibrosis.

Further reading

Alton EW, Geddes DM. Gene therapy for cystic fibrosis. *Eur Respir J* 1997; **10**: 257–9.

Davis PB. Evolution of therapy for cystic fibrosis. *N Engl J Med* 1994; **331**: 672–3.

Elborn JS, Shale DJ, Britton JR. Cystic fibrosis: current survival and population estimates to the year 2000. *Thorax* 1991; **46**: 881–5.

Hoiby N, Koch C. *Pseudomonas aeruginosa* infection in cystic fibrosis and its management. *Thorax* 1990; **45**: 881–4.

Stableforth DE, Smith DL. *Pseudomonas (Burkholderia) cepacia* in cystic fibrosis. *Thorax* 1994; **49**: 629–30.

CHAPTER 11

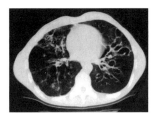

Asthma

Definition

Asthma is a disease characterized by **chronic airway inflammation** with **increased airway responsiveness** resulting in **symptoms** such as wheeze, cough and dyspnoea, and **airways obstruction** which is **variable** over short periods of time or **reversible** with treatment.

It is not a static uniform disease state but rather a **dynamic heterogenous clinical syndrome** which has a number of **different patterns** and which may progress through different stages so that not all features of the disease may be present in an individual patient at a particular point in time. For example, many patients with well controlled asthma are asymptomatic with normal lung function between attacks although if further investigations were performed there would usually be evidence of airway inflammation and increased airway responsiveness. By contrast, in some patients with chronic asthma the disease progresses to a state of irreversible airways obstruction. Some patients with smoking-related chronic obstructive pulmonary disease (COPD), bronchiectasis or cystic fibrosis may demonstrate airways obstruction with a degree of reversibility but it is important to appreciate that these diseases are different from asthma with distinct aetiologies, pathologies, natural history and responses to treatment.

Prevalence

Asthma has been recognized since ancient times and it is now estimated that 130 million people worldwide have asthma. The term is derived from the Greek word ασθμα, meaning short-drawn breath or panting and was in use in the time of Hippocrates (460–370 BC), although it was probably used to refer to many different causes of breathlessness. This problem of terminology continues in that the reported prevalence of asthma greatly depends on the criteria used to define asthma and is confused by changes in diagnostic habit (**labelling shift**) whereby patients may now be diagnosed as having asthma whereas previously they were labelled as having 'wheezy bronchitis' in the case of children or 'COPD' in the case of adults, for example. However, despite such labelling shifts there is a general consensus that the **prevalence of asthma is gradually increasing**. Studies using objective measures of reversible airways obstruction and airway hyperresponsiveness in combination with symptoms suggest that **about 7% of the adult population in the UK have asthma**. There is considerable interest in the reasons for the increasing prevalence of asthma and it is likely that such changes relate to environmental rather than genetic factors.

Aetiology (Fig. 11.1)

Asthma is multifactorial in origin arising from a

complex interaction of **genetic** and **environmental** factors. It seems likely that airway inflammation occurs when genetically susceptible individuals are exposed to certain environmental factors but the exact processes underlying asthma may vary from patient to patient. In many cases the most important environmental factors are the intensity, timing and mode of exposure to **aeroallergens** which stimulate the production of IgE. Additional environmental determinants are the concurrent exposure to **co-factors** such as cigarette smoke, atmospheric pollutants and respiratory tract infections.

Fig. 11.1 Asthma is multi-factorial in origin arising from a complex interaction of genetic and environmental factors, which result in airway inflammation and hyperresponsiveness, such that bronchoconstriction develops in response to a variety of trigger factors.

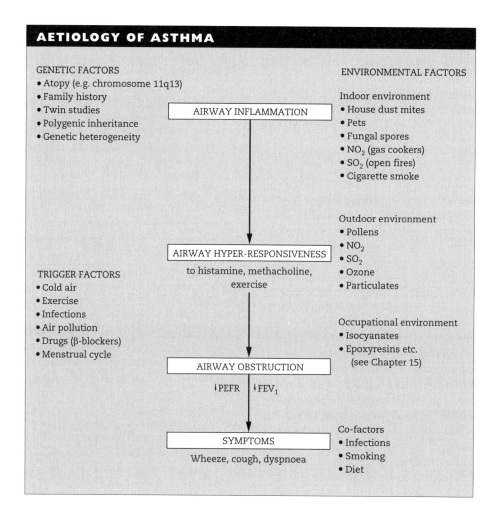

AETIOLOGY OF ASTHMA

GENETIC FACTORS
- Atopy (e.g. chromosome 11q13)
- Family history
- Twin studies
- Polygenic inheritance
- Genetic heterogeneity

AIRWAY INFLAMMATION

AIRWAY HYPER-RESPONSIVENESS
to histamine, methacholine, exercise

TRIGGER FACTORS
- Cold air
- Exercise
- Infections
- Air pollution
- Drugs (β-blockers)
- Menstrual cycle

AIRWAY OBSTRUCTION
↓PEFR   ↓FEV₁

SYMPTOMS
Wheeze, cough, dyspnoea

ENVIRONMENTAL FACTORS

Indoor environment
- House dust mites
- Pets
- Fungal spores
- NO₂ (gas cookers)
- SO₂ (open fires)
- Cigarette smoke

Outdoor environment
- Pollens
- NO₂
- SO₂
- Ozone
- Particulates

Occupational environment
- Isocyanates
- Epoxyresins etc.
  (see Chapter 15)

Co-factors
- Infections
- Smoking
- Diet

Genetic susceptibility

There is strong evidence of a hereditary contribution to the aetiology of asthma. It has long been known that asthma and atopy run in **families**. First-degree relatives of asthmatics have a significantly higher prevalence of asthma than relatives of non-asthmatic patients. It is important to appreciate, however, that families share environments as well as sharing genes, and that environmental factors are necessary for the expression of a genetic predisposition. **Atopy** is a constitutional tendency to produce significant amounts of IgE on exposure to small amounts of common antigens, Atopic individuals demonstrate positive reactions to antigens on skin prick tests and have a high prevalence of asthma, allergic rhinitis, urticaria and eczema. Several potential gene linkages (e.g. chromosome 11q13 location) to asthma and atopy have been suggested but it is clear that the genetic contribution to asthma is complex, possibly involving **polygenic inheritance** (several genes contributing to the asthmatic tendency in an individual) and **genetic heterogeneity** (different combinations of genes causing the asthmatic tendency in different individuals).

Environmental factors

The importance of environmental factors in the aetiology of asthma has been particularly evident in studies of populations who have **migrated from one country to another**. For example, children from the Pacific atoll of Tokelau were found to have developed asthma with similar prevalence to native New Zealand children when they were evacuated to New Zealand following a typhoon which devastated the local economy, whereas children remaining in Tokelau had a significantly lesser prevalence. It is likely that the increasing prevalence of asthma relates to environmental rather than genetic factors. There may be very many aspects of the environment which are important but a change to a **modern, urban, economically developed society seems to be particularly associated with the occurrence of asthma**.

Indoor environment

People spend at least 75% of their time indoors and overall exposure to air pollutants and allergens is determined more by concentrations indoors than outdoors. The indoor environment is particularly important in the case of young children since allergen exposure early in life may be particularly important in determining sensitization. There is a vast array of antigens in the typical home environment. **House dust mites** (*Dermatophagoides pteronyssius*) are found in high concentrations in carpets, soft furnishings and bedding. **Pet-derived allergens** are widespread in homes where dogs, cats or budgies are kept. **Feathers** are often present in pillows and duvets. Other antigens commonly present in homes are **fungal spores** and antigens from cockroaches. Pollutants such as **nitrogen dioxide** are commonly found at higher concentrations indoors than outside as a result of sources such as gas cookers and kerosene heaters. **Sulphur dioxide** and **particulate pollutants** are released from open fires or paraffin stoves. Passive exposure to **cigarette smoke** in the home has an adverse effect on asthma and other respiratory diseases in children in particular.

Outdoor environment

Although there is a widespread view among the general public that the increasing prevalence of asthma is attributable to atmospheric pollution from motor vehicles, the balance of evidence suggests that any such influence on the *initiation* of asthma is small. However, outdoor air quality plays an important, though complex and incompletely understood, role in *triggering exacerbations* of pre-existing asthma. Experimental and population studies have shown that nitrogen dioxide, ozone, sulphur dioxide and airborne particulates may have acute adverse effects on asthma during air pollution episodes.

* *Nitrogen dioxide (NO_2)*: the principal source of nitrogen dioxide and other nitrogen oxides (NO_x) is **motor vehicle emissions** but power stations and **fuel-burning industries**

also contribute. Nitrogen dioxide is also a common contaminant of indoor air arising from **gas cookers** and kerosene heaters. Nitrogen dioxide reacts with hydrocarbons and oxygen in the presence of sunlight, forming ozone. Emissions of nitrogen dioxide have increased over the last 30 years. Use of catalytic converters in cars reduces exhaust emissions.

• *Sulphur dioxide (SO$_2$)* is created by the **burning of fossil fuels** containing sulphur. **Power stations** are the main source of sulphur dioxide emissions although **domestic coal burning** is an important source in some areas. Diesel vehicles also emit sulphur dioxide. Levels of sulphur dioxide emissions are gradually declining.

• *Ozone (O$_3$)* is formed by a photochemical reaction involving sunlight, oxygen and nitrogen dioxide. Its production is dependent on **weather conditions**. Although nitrogen dioxide and sulphur dioxide levels tend to be higher in cities, ozone levels tend to be higher in rural areas.

• *Airborne particulates*: this is a term used to describe elements of **black smoke** consisting of small particles produced by incomplete combustion.

• *Antigens*: Levels of grass and flower **pollens** vary considerably depending on the climatic conditions and time of year, as do levels of **allergens** from rape seed, soy bean and other plants and crops.

Interactions between atmospheric pollutants, aeroallergens and climatic conditions have complex effects on asthma. Some studies suggest that exposure to **air pollution** may enhance airway responses to common **allergens**, thereby potentially playing a role in both the initiation of asthma and in the triggering of acute attacks. **Climatic conditions** such as high pressure and humidity with calm still air can result in an accumulation of airborne pollutants (e.g. particulates, ozone) and of allergens (e.g. pollens, fungal spores). Investigation of several epidemics of asthma in Barcelona in the 1980s established that the number of patients referred to hospital with acute attacks of asthma coincided with days when soybean was being unloaded from ships in the port in conditions of high barometric pressure and little wind. Several epidemics of acute asthma have been associated with thunderstorms, and these have particularly affected patients with pre-existing atopic asthma and IgE reactions to specific antigens such as pollens and fungal spores. Warm dry weather may cause a rapid rise in pollen concentrations and also in levels of O$_3$, nitrogen dioxide and sulphur dioxide because of atmospheric stability. Gusts of wind at the start of a thunderstorm lift allergens into the air. Rain disrupts pollen grains into a number of smaller allergenic particles. Under these circumstances atopic individuals with pre-existing asthma or hay fever are particularly vulnerable to the resultant allergen challenge. The effects of atmospheric pollutants and allergens on asthmatics is influenced by factors such as use of asthma medication, time spent outdoors and exercise (which increases ventilation).

Work environment
Many agents encountered in the workplace may induce **occupational asthma**, e.g. isocyanates, epoxyresins, persulphates, hard wood dusts (see Chapter 15).

Co-factors in asthma
A number of other factors influence the development of asthma.

• *Infections*: many respiratory infections (e.g. influenza A, *Mycoplasma pneumoniae*, *Chlamydia pneumoniae*) provoke a transient increase in airway responsiveness in normal individuals and in asthmatics. Conversely there is some evidence that viral infections (e.g. measles) in the first year of life may protect against asthma.

• *Smoking*: cigarette **smoking** is associated with increased levels of IgE and with increased sensitization to certain occupational allergens in particular (e.g. anhydrides). **Maternal smoking** during pregnancy is thought to increase the risk of developing atopic disease in infancy and **passive exposure** to smoking has an adverse effect on asthma and other respiratory diseases.

• *Diet*: some studies suggest that **breast feeding** may offer protection against the subsequent development of asthma possibly because of reduced exposure to food allergens in the neonatal period. Airway responsiveness may be influenced by dietary **salt intake** although studies show conflicting results. In some patients asthmatic attacks may occasionally be precipitated by certain foods such as milk, egg, wheat and food **additives** and preservatives (e.g. tartrazine). Diets high in **oily fish** appear to be protective.

• Drugs: β-**blocking drugs** can induce bronchoconstriction in asthmatics, sometimes even when given in eye drops (e.g. timolol for glaucoma). A small percentage of asthmatics develop bronchoconstriction when given **salicylates** (e.g. aspirin) or **non-steroidal anti-inflammatory drugs** (e.g. ibuprofen). These drugs block arachidonic acid metabolism down the prostaglandin pathway diverting it to the leukotriene pathway. A reaction to aspirin is more common in asthmatics with nasal polyps.

Pathogenesis and pathology (Fig. 11.2)

A series of factors combine to produce increasing airway inflammation and airway responsiveness, and when these features reach a sufficient level bronchoconstriction and asthma symptoms are triggered. Typically, the inhalation of an allergen in a sensitized atopic asthmatic results in a two-phase response consisting of an **early asthmatic reaction** reaching its maximum at about 20 minutes, and a **late asthmatic reaction** developing about 6–12 hours later. These atopic asthmatics have high levels of specific IgE which binds to receptors on inflammatory cells, most notably mast cells. Interaction of the IgE antibody and inhaled antigen results in the activation of these inflammatory cells and release of pre-formed mediators such as histamine, prostaglandins and leukotrienes which cause contraction of smooth muscle of the airways producing bronchoconstriction. The inflammatory response in asthma is highly complex

Fig. 11.2 Summary of the pathological features of asthma. Half of a cross-section of a bronchiole is shown. Although these features are characteristic of appearances after death from asthma, identical appearances are present patchily in patients who are apparently untroubled by their asthma at the time.

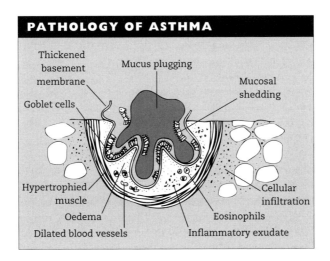

PATHOLOGY OF ASTHMA

Thickened basement membrane
Mucus plugging
Mucosal shedding
Goblet cells
Hypertrophied muscle
Cellular infiltration
Oedema
Eosinophils
Dilated blood vessels
Inflammatory exudate

involving the full **spectrum of inflammatory cells** including mast cells, eosinophils, B and T lymphocytes and neutrophils, which release an **array of mediators and cytokines**. These mediators regulate the response of other inflammatory cells, and have a number of effects resulting in **contraction of airway smooth muscle, increased vascular permeability** and stimulation of airway **mucus secretion**. T-helper lymphocytes have an important role in the regulation of the inflammatory response. These cells may be divided into two main subsets on the basis of the profile of cytokines which they produce. **Th2 cells** produce interleukin 4 (IL-4), IL-5, IL-6 and IL-10 and **up-regulate** the specific form of airway inflammation of asthma by enhancing IgE synthesis and eosinophil and mast-cell function. In contrast **Th1 cells** produce IL-2, interferon γ (IFN-γ) and lymphotoxin and **down-regulate the atopic response**. In those who are genetically susceptible to developing asthma, antigen presentation to T-helper cells leads to a Th2 response. Infection with respiratory syncytial virus augments a Th2 response whereas some other microbial antigens lead to a Th1 response. It has been suggested that exposure to allergens and infections in early childhood is important in determining the pattern of immune response thereby modulating the genetic susceptibility to developing asthma.

The wall of the airway in asthma is thickened by oedema, cellular infiltration, increased smooth-muscle mass and glands (Fig. 11.1). With increasing severity and chronicity of the disease **remodelling of the airway** occurs leading to fibrosis of the airway wall, fixed narrowing of the airway and a reduced response to bronchodilator medication. Mucus plugging of the lumen of the airway is a prominent feature of acute severe asthma. Although in clinical practice patients with asthma are sometimes classified as having extrinsic asthma (occurring in relation to inhalation of environmental antigens) or intrinsic asthma (occurring without any definable relationship to an environmental antigen) the pathological features of

the airway inflammation are identical. It is likely that the inflammatory cascade of asthma can be initiated by a variety of different factors in different patients.

Clinical features

The typical symptoms of asthma are **wheeze, dyspnoea, cough** and a sensation of **'chest tightness'**. These symptoms may occur for the first time at any age and may be episodic or persistent. In **episodic asthma** the patient is often asymptomatic between episodes but suffers attacks of asthma during viral respiratory tract infections or after exposure to certain allergens. This pattern of asthma is commonly seen in children and young adults who are **atopic** and sensitized to common antigens (e.g. grass pollens, pet dander). Because episodes of asthma can often be related to inhaled environmental antigens the clinical term **'extrinsic asthma'** is occasionally used. Sometimes the clinical pattern is of **persistent asthma** with chronic wheeze and dyspnoea. This pattern is more common in older patients with **'adult-onset'** asthma who are non-atopic and whose symptoms are not related to any apparent antigen exposure so that the term **'intrinsic asthma'** is sometimes used. The variable nature of symptoms is a characteristic feature of asthma. Typically there is a diurnal pattern (Fig. 11.3) with symptoms and peak expiratory flow measurements being worse early in the morning — so-called **'morning dipping'**. Symptoms such as cough and wheeze often disturb sleep and the term **'nocturnal asthma'** emphasizes this. Cough is often the dominant symptom and the lack of wheeze or dyspnoea may lead to a delay in making the diagnosis: so-called, **'cough variant asthma'**. Symptoms may be provoked by exercise: **'exercise asthma'**. These descriptive clinical terms are useful in emphasizing some characteristic features of asthma, and highlight the fact that asthma is not a uniform, static disease but a broad, dynamic clinical syndrome.

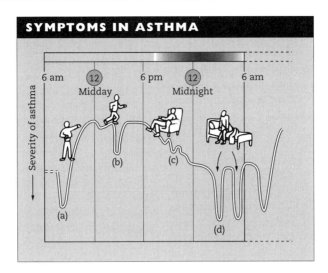

SYMPTOMS IN ASTHMA

Fig. 11.3 Diurnal variation in symptoms in asthma. The most striking features are usually: (a) chest tightness and wheezing dyspnoea on waking, improving during the morning and (d) nocturnal attacks. In addition there may be exercise-induced asthma (b) and worsening of symptoms whilst resting in the evening (c).

When assessing a patient with confirmed or suspected asthma it is important to focus on key aspects of the history which not only aid diagnosis but which are also important in assessing the pattern of the asthma and in treatment.

• *Family history*: there is a significantly increased prevalence of asthma in relatives of patients with asthma or other atopic diseases (eczema, hay fever).

• *Home environment*: smoking, or exposure to passive smoking in the home environment, is an adverse factor. Indoor allergens, e.g. house dust mite, dog or cat dander may be important in triggering attacks.

• *Occupational history*: it is important to identify if the patient's asthma could have been caused by exposure to asthmagenic agents at work, by enquiring about current and previous jobs, the tasks performed and materials used. Do symptoms improve away from work at weekends or on holidays? Are symptoms worse on return to work, particularly the evening or night after work? (See Chapter 15.)

• *Trigger factors*: are there any factors which precipitate symptoms?

   (a) Exercise.

   (b) Cold air.

   (c) Viral respiratory infections.

   (d) Allergen exposure (e.g. feather pillows, cat dander).

   (e) Seasonal factors (e.g. grass pollen).

   (f) Drugs (e.g. β-blockers, aspirin).

• *Response to treatment*: enquiry about the effectiveness of previous treatment with bronchodilator drugs or prednisolone yields clues to the reversibility of the disease and is particularly important in detecting asthma in older patients who may have been erroneously labelled as having COPD.

The characteristic features on examination of patients with asthma are diffuse bilateral **wheeze** (rhonchi) and a **prolonged expiratory phase** to respiration, but there are often no signs detectable between episodes. There may be features of associated diseases such as allergic rhinitis, nasal polyps and eczema. It is essential to be alert for atypical features such as unilateral wheeze which suggests local bronchial obstruction by a foreign body (e.g.

inhaled peanut) in a child or a carcinoma in an adult, for example. It is also important to ensure that there are no signs of cardiac or other respiratory disease. During acute attacks of asthma features such as tachycardia, tachypnoea, cyanosis, use of accessory muscles of respiration and features of anxiety and general distress indicate a severe episode. Pulsus paradoxus (a fall of more than 10 mmHg in systolic blood pressure during inspiration) may be present but is an unreliable indicator of severity. Chronic severe childhood asthma may cause chest deformity with the sternum being pushed forwards (pigeon chest deformity) and the lower rib cage being pulled inwards (Harrison's sulci) (Fig. 11.4).

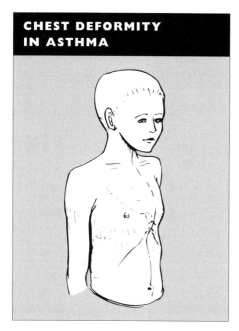

CHEST DEFORMITY IN ASTHMA

Fig. 11.4 Chest deformity in chronic childhood asthma. The sternum is pushed forwards (pigeon chest deformity) and there is a groove approximately in the position of the sixth rib (Harrison's sulcus). Deformity of the type shown is always indicative of severe asthma. It is, to a considerable extent, reversible if asthma is treated adequately and sufficiently early. It should be a rarity. (Original drawing reproduced by kind permission of Dr R.A.L. Brewis. From *Lecture Notes on Respiratory Disease*, 1st edn.)

Investigations

Lung function tests

The key feature of asthma is airways obstruction which is variable over short periods of time or reversible with treatment. Measurement of airways obstruction using a peak expiratory flow meter or spirometer is as essential in assessing a patient with asthma as measurement of blood pressure using a sphygmomanometer is in a patient with hypertension.

• *Airways obstruction*: peak expiratory flow, forced expiratory volume in 1 second (FEV_1) and FEV_1/vital capacity (VC) ratio are reduced in active asthma. However, asthma is a dynamic condition and peak flow and spirometry may be normal between attacks in a patient with episodic asthma.

• *Reversibility* (Fig. 11.5): if airways obstruction is detected by peak flow or spirometry the next step is to assess its reversibility to **bronchodilator drugs**. Typically, the patient is given 200 µg of salbutamol and spirometry or peak flow measurements are repeated 15–20 minutes later. Patients with active asthma characteristically show airways obstruction with a large bronchodilator response. Patients with more severe chronic asthma may fail to show an improvement after a bronchodilator drug but demonstrate reversibility to **steroids**. A therapeutic trial of prednisolone 30 mg/day for 14 days often results in a marked improvement in airways obstruction in patients who have failed to show reversibility to bronchodilator drugs.

• *Variability* (Fig. 11.5): the variability of the airways obstruction of asthma is demonstrated by **serial measurements of peak flow** or spirometry over a period of time. The patient is given a peak flow meter and taught to record measurements four times daily. A characteristic pattern is '**morning dipping**' in which peak flow values are lowest in the morning, improving throughout the day. This diurnal variability is most marked in active, poorly controlled asthma. Serial peak flow measurements may

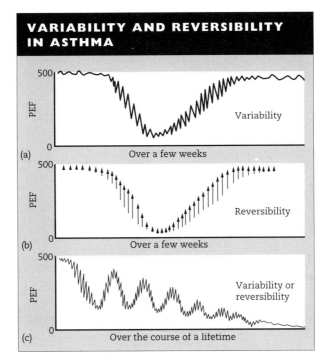

VARIABILITY AND REVERSIBILITY IN ASTHMA

(a) Variability — Over a few weeks

(b) Reversibility — Over a few weeks

(c) Variability or reversibility — Over the course of a lifetime

Fig. 11.5 Variability and reversibility in asthma—three diagrammatic views. (a) In the course of an exacerbation and subsequent recovery, variability (diurnal variation) is most marked when asthma is moderately severe and may be absent when asthma is either very mild or very severe. (b) In the course of an exacerbation and subsequent recovery, reversibility after an inhaled bronchodilator (arrows) is most marked when asthma is moderately severe and may be absent when asthma is either very mild or very severe. (c) Over decades of chronic asthma, there is a general tendency for a decline in overall ventilatory performance, which is related to the duration and severity of the earlier experience. Accompanying this there is a reduction in both variability and reversibility.

also be used to demonstrate the variability of airways obstruction in relation to factors such as exercise or environmental allergens, for example.

Total lung capacity is usually increased in asthma as a manifestation of **hyperinflation**, and residual volume is elevated indicating **air trapping**. In contrast to patients with COPD (see Chapter 12) the airways obstruction of asthma is not associated with any impairment of gas diffusion so that transfer factor for carbon monoxide ($T_L co$) and transfer co-efficient ($K co$) are characteristically normal or indeed slightly elevated. During an acute severe attack of asthma, **hypoxaemia** devel-ops and is usually associated with increased ventilation and a reduced $P co_2$. Elevation of $P co_2$ in a patient with asthma is a sign of a critically ill patient who is failing to maintain ventilation.

Airway responsiveness

Airway responsiveness is a measure of the general **'irritability' of the airways**, the degree to which **bronchoconstriction develops in response to physical or chemical stimuli**.

• *Exercise testing*: one of the most useful ways of demonstrating increased airway responsive-ness or hyperreactivity is to measure peak flow or spirometry before and after 5–10 minutes of vigorous exercise. A post-exercise fall in FEV_1 or peak flow of more than 10% is highly suggestive of asthma, as normal subjects usually show a degree of bronchodilatation, rather than bronchoconstriction, during exercise. An **exercise provocation test** is most useful if a patient with suspected asthma has normal peak flow or spirometry when seen in the clinic, such that reversibility testing may be of little use, and a 'provocation' test is more useful. The response is greater if exercise is performed in cold air.

• *Histamine/methacholine provocation tests*: the degree of airway responsiveness can be measured precisely in the laboratory. Under careful supervision the patient inhales increasing doses of nebulized **histamine** or **methacholine**, starting at a very low dose, and serial spirometry is performed. By plotting the percentage fall in FEV_1 the concentration (C), or dose (D), of the chemical provoking (P) a 20% fall in FEV_1, can be calculated and expressed as a figure, e.g. PD_{20} methacholine 200 μg or PC_{20} histamine 4 mg/ml. Histamine or methacholine provocation tests are not usually required for the diagnosis of asthma in routine practice but are particularly useful in assessing changes in airway responsiveness in relation to exposure to environmental or occupational allergens (see Chapter 15), and in research studies.

Tests for hypersensitivity

Skin prick tests (Fig. 11.6) may be performed to identify atopy and to detect particular sensitivity to a specific antigen with a view to exclusion of exposure where possible (e.g. cat allergens). Drops of antigen extracts are placed on the flexor surface of the forearm and the tip of a small stylet is pressed into the superficial epidermis through the drop of allergen. A positive reaction is manifest as a weal with a surrounding erythematous flare at about 15 minutes. The reaction to allergens should be compared with the reaction to a drop of histamine and to a drop of control solution containing no antigens. Total **IgE level** is often elevated in patients with atopic asthma and they sometimes have a mild peripheral blood **eosinophilia. RAST testing** (radioallergosorbent test) is a means of measuring the level of circulating IgE specifically directed towards a particular antigen.

Some asthmatics develop an allergic reaction to *Aspergillus fumigatus*, a ubiquitous fungus which may colonize the airways. In these cir-

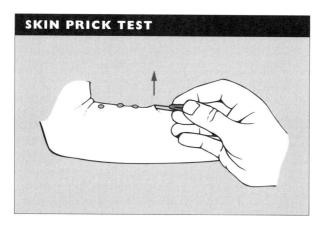

SKIN PRICK TEST

Fig. 11.6 Skin prick test. Drops of antigen extracts and antigen-free control solution are placed on the flexor surface of the forearm. Each drop is pricked with a fine needle. The needle is held parallel to the skin surface, advanced slightly and a tiny fold of skin lifted briefly as shown. Deep stabs and bleeding should be avoided. Weal and flare are measured after 10–20 minutes. Vigorous preparation of the skin is undesirable.

cumstances the asthma is typically severe and persistent requiring systemic steroid treatment. There is often associated severe airway inflammation and mucus plugging resulting in bronchiectasis (see Chapter 9). In addition to a positive skin prick test to *Aspergillus* these patients often have significant eosinophilia and **precipitating antibodies to Aspergillus** in their serum. Very rarely asthma occurs as part of an eosinophilic vasculitis such as Churg–Strauss syndrome (see Chapter 16) in which case very high levels of blood eosinophilia occur.

General investigations

Further general investigations may be necessary to exclude other cardiorespiratory diseases. **Chest X-ray** is essential in older patients who have smoked, to exclude bronchial carcinoma, for example, and may be needed in children if there are any clinical features to suggest other diseases such as cystic fibrosis or bronchiectasis. **Bronchoscopy** is occasionally necessary to assess for vocal cord dysfunction, inhaled foreign bodies, bronchial

carcinoma or rarer causes of bronchial obstruction such as carcinoid tumours.

Diagnosis (Table 11.1)

Although diagnosing asthma is straightforward when the patient presents with classic symptoms and evidence of variable or reversible airways obstruction, there are many pitfalls, and errors in diagnosis are common. **Failure to diagnose** asthma results in the patient being deprived of appropriate asthma treatment, e.g. a child with cough receiving recurrent courses of antibiotics for 'chest infections' when in fact he is suffering from cough variant asthma. Conversely **incorrect diagnosis** of asthma might expose the patient to the risks of inappropriate treatment (e.g. recurrent courses of prednisolone) and delay appropriate management of other lung disease, e.g. inhaled foreign body in a child or tracheal tumour in an adult producing **wheeze simulating asthma**. On the one hand it is necessary to be alert to less well recognized presentations of

---

DIAGNOSING ASTHMA

Underdiagnosis: Could this patient's symptoms be due to asthma?
Overdiagnosis: Does this patient really have asthma?

- Recognize **symptoms** suggestive of asthma, e.g. wheeze, cough, recurrent 'chest infections'

- Establish evidence of **airways obstruction**, e.g. ↓ peak flow, ↓FEV_1, ↓FEV_1/VC ratio

- Assess **variability**, **reversibility**, **provocability** of airway obstruction: serial peak flow chart, e.g. morning dipping; response to bronchodilator and steroid trial; exercise-induced fall in peak flow

- **Monitor** progress and **review diagnosis**, e.g. has 'wheezy bronchitis' of childhood evolved into established asthma or was it due to viral bronchiolitis?

- Consider **additional diagnoses**, e.g. occupational asthma, allergic bronchopulmonary aspergillosis

- Exclude **alternative diagnoses**
  Children: e.g. inhaled foreign body, cystic fibrosis
  Adults: e.g. bronchial carcinoma, cardiac failure, COPD

COPD, chronic obstructive pulmonary disease; FEV_1, forced expiratory volume in 1 second; VC, vital capacity.

Table 11.1 Diagnosing asthma.

asthma, e.g. cough without wheeze, and on the other hand to be prepared to review the evidence for asthma if the response to treatment is poor or if unusual features emerge (e.g. could this child possibly have cystic fibrosis?). Evidence establishing the diagnosis of asthma and excluding other diseases often emerges over time and it is sometimes wise to use interim terms such as **'suspected asthma'** while gathering evidence of variable or reversible airways obstruction that allows a **firm diagnosis** of asthma to be established. Doubt may arise where it is difficult to obtain accurate peak flow or spirometry measurements as in the case of young children. Even when the diagnosis of asthma is established the diagnostic process should be taken further: **could this be occupational asthma?** Is there evidence of additional lung disease such as bronchiectasis or allergic bronchopulmonary aspergillosis? The doctor needs to exercise good clinical skills in applying two critical questions: **could this patient's symptoms be due to asthma? Does this patient really have asthma?**

Management (Fig. 11.7)

Patient education

Successful management of asthma requires that the **patient**, or the **parents** of a child, with asthma understand the nature of the condition and its treatment. Patient education should begin at the time of diagnosis and form part of every subsequent consultation between the patient and **doctor**. All members of the **team** should participate in the process and there is a particular role for respiratory **nurse specialists**.

Education involves the patient understanding the **nature of asthma**, learning the **practical skills** necessary to manage asthma and adopting the appropriate actions in managing their asthma and **adhering to treatment**. Education of the patient often starts with a discussion of the multi-factorial aetiology of asthma and identification of **precipitating factors**. It is useful for patients to understand that inflammation of the airways is a key factor underlying the development of wheeze as they can then appreciate the difference between **'reliever'** (**bronchodilator**) and **'preventer'** (**anti-inflammatory**) medication. Sufficient time should be invested in instructing the patient in the **use of inhaler devices**, as this is a crucial aspect determining the effectiveness of prescribed medication.

Use of a **peak flow meter** provides patients with an objective measure of airway obstruction allowing them to see the variability of readings from day to day, the influence of precipitating factors and the effect of treatment. Most patients with asthma should be able to **monitor and manage** their asthma themselves to a considerable degree and to recognize when medical advice is needed, in much the same way as patients with diabetes monitor their blood sugar levels and adjust insulin therapy.

The amount of information given to each patient needs to be varied in accordance with their needs and aptitude but all patients should know about features which indicate when their asthma is deteriorating and what action to take in these circumstances. Doctors should be aware that it is often those patients least interested in learning about their disease who are at greatest risk and that features such as depression, anxiety, denial of disease and non-compliance with treatment are strongly associated with asthma deaths. Particular effort is required to identify and target resources at such patients. Information conveyed in discussion with the patient should be supplemented by **personalized written information**. Many patients are frightened and anxious about the diagnosis of asthma and it is often helpful to point out that many top-class sports men and women have asthma which does not impair their performance. Many such sports people lend their support to organizations such as the National Asthma Campaign in the UK which provide literature and support to help patients with asthma.

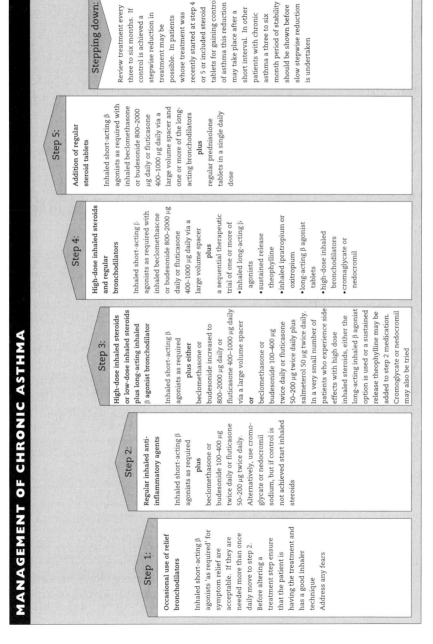

MANAGEMENT OF CHRONIC ASTHMA

Step 1:

Occasional use of relief bronchodilators

Inhaled short-acting β agonists 'as required' for symptom relief are acceptable. If they are needed more than once daily move to step 2.
Before altering a treatment step ensure that the patient is having the treatment and has a good inhaler technique
Address any fears

Step 2:

Regular inhaled anti-inflammatory agents

Inhaled short-acting β agonists as required
plus
beclomethasone or budesonide 100–400 μg twice daily or fluticasone 50–200 μg twice daily.
Alternatively, use cromoglycate or nedocromil sodium, but if control is not achieved start inhaled steroids

Step 3:

High-dose inhaled steroids or low-dose inhaled steroids plus long-acting inhaled β agonist bronchodilator

Inhaled short-acting β agonists as required
plus either
beclomethasone or budesonide increased to 800–2000 μg daily or fluticasone 400–1000 μg daily via a large volume spacer
or
beclomethasone or budesonide 100–400 μg twice daily or fluticasone 50–200 μg twice daily plus salmeterol 50 μg twice daily. In a very small number of patients who experience side effects with high dose inhaled steroids, either the long-acting inhaled β agonist option is used or a sustained release theophylline may be added to step 2 medication. Cromoglycate or nedocromil may also be tried

Step 4:

High-dose inhaled steroids and regular bronchodilators

Inhaled short-acting β agonists as required with inhaled beclomethasone or budesonide 800–2000 μg daily or fluticasone 400–1000 μg daily via a large volume spacer
plus
a sequential therapeutic trial of one or more of
• inhaled long-acting β agonists
• sustained release theophylline
• inhaled ipratropium or oxitropium
• long-acting β agonist tablets
• high-dose inhaled bronchodilators
• cromoglycate or nedocromil

Step 5:

Addition of regular steroid tablets

Inhaled short-acting β agonists as required with inhaled beclomethasone or budesonide 800–2000 μg daily or fluticasone 400–1000 μg daily via a large volume spacer and one or more of the long-acting bronchodilators
plus
regular prednisolone tablets in a single daily dose

Stepping down:

Review treatment every three to six months. If control is achieved a stepwise reduction in treatment may be possible. In patients whose treatment was recently started at step 4 or 5 or included steroid tablets for gaining control of asthma this reduction may take place after a short interval. In other patients with chronic asthma a three to six month period of stability should be shown before slow stepwise reduction is undertaken

Fig. 11.7 Management of chronic asthma. (Reproduced with permission from British Thoracic Society guidelines on asthma management. Thorax 1997; **52** (suppl. I).)

Avoidance of precipitating factors

Most patients with atopic asthma react to many different antigens so that environmental control measures are generally not particularly helpful. **House dust mites** are most prevalent in warm moist areas containing desquamated human skin scales and they are almost universally distributed in mattresses, pillows, carpets, furnishings and soft toys. The level of house dust mite may be reduced by encasing mattresses in occlusive covers and by frequent washing of blankets and duvets. Humidity levels can be decreased by better ventilation. Avoidance of exposure to **pet allergens** from dogs or cats, for example, is more feasible but the result of these interventions is often disappointing. Similarly it is difficult to avoid exposure to **outdoor allergens** but some patients benefit from precautions such as increasing asthma treatment or remaining indoors with closed windows when pollen counts are high.

Desensitization (immunotherapy) is a highly specialized technique in which repeated injections of an allergen are given to a sensitized subject in an attempt to produce 'blocking antibody' of IgG type which prevents the allergen binding to specific IgE on mast cells. It is most commonly used in the treatment of well documented life-threatening anaphylactic reactions to insect stings but there is little evidence of its benefit in asthma and any potential benefit does not justify the risk of provoking a major allergic reaction.

Avoidance of irritants such as **cigarette smoke** or generally dusty environments is advisable. **Avoidance of β-blocker** drugs is important for all patients with asthma, and patients who are sensitive to **aspirin** should avoid all aspirin-containing products and non-steroidal anti-inflammatory drugs. **Viral infections** often precipitate attacks of asthma so that it is advisable for patients to monitor peak flow measurements carefully during such infections and to intensify asthma treatment as required. Since influenza infection may precipitate severe exacerbations of asthma, annual **influenza vaccination** is recommended.

Exercise is a particular factor precipitating asthma. Bronchoconstriction may develop within minutes of onset of vigorous activity. This response usually resolves within 30 minutes and there then follows a refractory period of about 2 hours when further exercise does not provoke bronchoconstriction. Therefore a warm-up period before the main exercise usually controls this problem. Use of β-agonist medication or sodium cromoglycate before exercise usually prevents exercise induced asthma, allowing athletes with asthma to compete at the highest level of their sport. For example, 67 athletes at the 1984 Olympic Games had asthma, and many won medals!

Drug treatment

Bronchodilator drugs ('relievers') are used to relieve symptoms of bronchoconstriction. **Anti-inflammatory drugs ('preventers')** treat the underlying chronic inflammatory process in asthma. Short courses of oral **prednisolone ('rescue medication')** are used to treat exacerbations. Most patients with chronic asthma can be managed very satisfactorily with regular inhaled steroids to control airway inflammation, an inhaled bronchodilator to be taken as required to reverse wheezing, and training to initiate emergency prednisolone treatment when needed.

Bronchodilators

• $β_2$-agonists: (e.g. salbutamol, terbutaline) stimulate β-adrenoceptors in the smooth muscle of the airway, producing smooth-muscle relaxation and **bronchodilatation**. They have an onset of action within 15 minutes and a duration of action of 4–6 hours. Side-effects include tremor, palpitations and muscle cramps but these are uncommon unless high doses are used. The main concern about bronchodilator medication is that over-reliance on these drugs may disguise the severity of the asthma by providing symptom relief but not control of the underlying inflammatory process (in much the same way as a pain-killer relieves pain but does not treat the cause).

Increasing need for bronchodilator medication is an indication of poorly controlled asthma and a need to increase anti-inflammatory medication.

• *Long-acting β-agonists*: (e.g. salmeterol, formoterol) have a duration of action of more than 12 hours and are particularly helpful in **controlling nocturnal symptoms**. Their use is only recommended as an adjunct to inhaled corticosteroids so that control of the airway inflammation is not neglected.

• *Anti-cholinergic bronchodilators*: (e.g. ipratropium, oxitropium) produce bronchodilatation by **blocking the bronchoconstrictor effect of vagal nerve** stimulation on bronchial smooth muscle. They take about 1 hour to reach their maximum effect and have a duration of action of about 4–6 hours. Side-effects are uncommon but nebulized anti-cholinergic drugs may be deposited in the eyes, aggravating glaucoma. In most patients with asthma they are less effective than $β_2$-agonists but they may be useful in young children and older patients.

• *Theophyllines* increase cyclic adenosine monophosphate (AMP) stimulation of β-adrenoceptors by **inhibiting the metabolism of cyclic AMP** by the enzyme phosphodiesterase. They may also have other effects including some anti-inflammatory actions. They are not available in inhaler form and absorption from the gastrointestinal tract and clearance of the drug by the liver are variable so that the dose needs to be titrated carefully in accordance with blood levels. Side-effects such as nausea, vomiting, headache, tachycardia and malaise, are common. Hepatic clearance of theophyllines is reduced by drugs such as cimetidine, ciprofloxacin and erythromycin, and toxicity can occur if these medications are prescribed without adjustment in the dose of theophylline. Aminophylline is an intravenous form of theophylline (combined with ethylenediamine for solubility) which may be used in severe attacks of asthma not responding to β-agonist medication. It must be given slowly (over at least 20 minutes) with careful adjustment of dose in accordance with blood levels in order to avoid serious toxicity such as convulsions and cardiac arrhythmias.

Anti-inflammatory drugs

• *Inhaled corticosteroids* (e.g. beclomethasone, budesonide, fluticasone) are the mainstay of asthma treatment since they **counteract airway inflammation** which is the key underlying process in asthma. It is essential that the patient understands that this is a **preventative treatment** which needs to be taken regularly and which does not provide immediate relief of symptoms. **Compliance** is improved by using a twice-daily regimen whereby the patient's 'preventative' steroid inhaler is left at their bedside and taken regularly every night and morning whereas their 'reliever' bronchodilator is carried around with them for use as required. The dose is adjusted to give optimal control and varies greatly from patient to patient. Many adult patients with relatively mild asthma achieve good control with a dose of about 400 μg beclomethasone per day, but some patients with chronic severe asthma may require 2000 μg per day. In adult patients **'low-dose'** (below the equivalent of about 1000 μg beclomethasone per day) inhaled steroids are not usually associated with any significant side-effects apart from oropharyngeal candidiasis or hoarseness of the voice which can be reduced by using a spacer device and gargling the throat with water after inhalation. With **'high dose'** inhaled steroids (above about 1000 μg beclomethasone per day) biochemical evidence of suppression of adrenal function, and increased bone turnover are detectable in some patients. The clinical significance of such systemic effects needs to be considered in the context of the dangers of uncontrolled asthma and alternative therapies such as oral prednisolone. The dosage of inhaled steroids should be reviewed regularly to ensure that the patient is taking as much as is required to control their asthma ('step up') but, equally as little as necessary ('step down') so as to minimize the risk of side-effects with long-term usage.

• *Sodium cromoglycate* is a preventative inhaled treatment which has a number of anti-inflammatory action including stabilization of mast cells. It is mainly used in children with mild asthma and it has no significant side-effects. However, it is less effective than inhaled steroids in more troublesome asthma. Nedocromil is a newer inhaled compound with similar properties to cromoglycate.

• *Oral steroid treatment*: **'rescue' courses** of oral steroids may be needed to control exacerbations of asthma. Typically this consists of prednisolone 30–40 mg/day for about 7–14 days in an adult. Treatment is continued until asthma control has been achieved. Most patients should be taught to start their own short course of oral prednisolone in accordance with a predetermined self-management plan: e.g. when peak flow falls below 60% of the patient's best value. Patients should understand the potential side-effects of long-term use of prednisolone and the difference between this and infrequent short-course usage which is safe. A very small number of patients require **long-term systemic prednisolone** to control severe asthma. These patients should be attending a hospital specialist and it should have been clearly established that their asthma cannot be controlled by other measures. The dose of steroids needs to be kept as low as possible. In these circumstances the patient should be given a **'steroid treatment card'** documenting the dose of steroids used, advising about side-effects and warning patients that steroids should not be stopped suddenly because of the risk of adrenal insufficiency. Booster doses may be required during illnesses and patients may be particularly susceptible to infections such as chickenpox: other **adverse effects** include peptic ulceration, myopathy, osteoporosis, growth suppression, depression, psychosis, cataracts, and cushingoid features. Patients receiving long-term oral prednisolone should be considered for preventative treatment of osteoporosis such as smoking cessation, exercise, hormone replacement therapy, adequate dietary calcium intake and disodium etidronate/calcium treatment where appropriate.

Stepwise approach to treatment of asthma

The British Thoracic Society guidelines on the management of asthma recommend a stepwise approach to treatment according to the severity of the asthma in order to gain control of the disease. The aims of treatment are to abolish symptoms, to restore normal or best possible airway function and to reduce the risk of severe attacks as much as possible. Patients should start treatment at the step most appropriate to the initial severity of their asthma and treatment is adjusted as appropriate thereafter. For the majority of patients asthma is controlled by a combination of a regular inhaled steroid and use of an inhaled bronchodilator drug as required. Bronchodilator drugs are primarily intended to provide symptom relief whereas inhaled steroids are targeted at the underlying inflammatory process in the airways. Treatment should be **'stepped up' as much as necessary** to control the asthma; when control has been achieved treatment may be **'stepped down'** so that the patient is on **no more treatment than is necessary**.

Asthma is a dynamic condition changing over time and ongoing management requires an assessment of the level of control of the asthma that has been achieved and adjustment of medication to find the optimal balance between control of the asthma, use of medication, and potential side-effects of treatment. **Assessing asthma control** involves:

• measurement of peak flow or spirometry and comparing the values with the patient's best value and predicted normal value;

• monitoring of serial peak flow records over several days to assess diurnal and day-to-day variability;

• assessment of the patient's requirements for use of bronchodilator 'reliever' medication and 'rescue' courses of oral steroids;

• noting absences from work or school because of asthma;

• assessment of level of symptoms, e.g. noc-

PRESSURIZED METERED DOSE INHALER

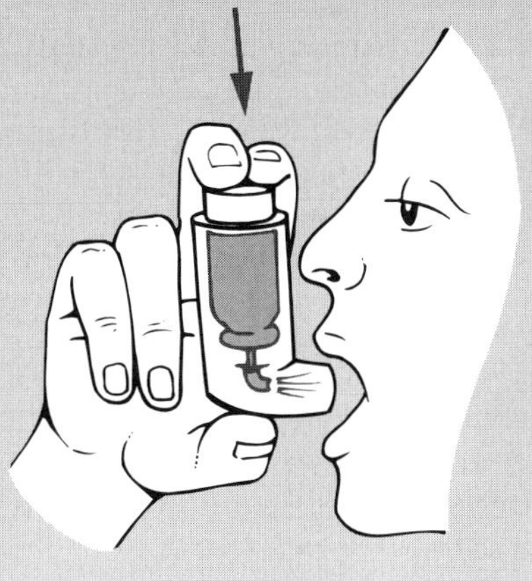

- Remove the cap and shake the inhaler
- Tilt the head back slightly and exhale
- Position the inhaler in the mouth (or preferably just in front of the open mouth)
- During a slow inspiration, press down the inhaler to release the medication
- Continue inhalation to full inspiration
- Hold breath for 10 seconds
- Actuate only one puff per inhalation

Fig. 11.8 Pressurized metered dose inhaler.

turnal sleep disturbance or exercise-induced bronchospasm.

Inhaler devices

The inhaled route is preferred for β-agonists and corticosteroids since it allows these drugs to be delivered directly to the airway reducing the risk of systemic side-effects. A variety of inhaler devices are available.

• *Metered dose inhalers* (Fig. 11.8): pressurized metered dose inhalers were first introduced in 1956 and use chlorofluorocarbons (CFCs) as a propellant. **CFCs damage the ozone layer** and in 1987 the Montreal Protocol was enacted under the auspices of the United Nations environmental programme committing governments to the phasing out of CFCs, including their use in aerosol inhalers, by about the year 2000. A number of propellant-free dry-powder devices are already available and some CFC-free metered dose inhalers using hydrofluoroalkane (HFA) are being developed. It is essential to instruct the patient in the correct use of the inhaler (Fig. 11.8) and this should be rechecked frequently. About 10% of the drug is delivered to the lower airways and the remainder is mainly deposited in the oropharynx and swallowed into the gastrointestinal tract where it is absorbed into the blood, but mostly metabolized by first-pass metabolism in the liver.

• *Spacer devices* (Fig. 11.9): poor inhaler technique is a significant problem in the use of metered dose inhalers. Large-volume spacer devices overcome some of these problems and improve deposition of the drugs in the lower airway to about 20% on average. The canister (cr) of pressurized aerosol is inserted into one end of the spacer device and the patient breathes through the other end via a one-way valve (v) which closes on expiration; (e) expiratory port. This **reduces the need for coordination of inspiration and activation of the inhaler**. Distancing the inhaler from the mouth ('spacing') results in a fine aerosol of smaller particles **improving delivery of the drug to the lower airways**.

• *Dry-powder devices* (Fig. 11.10): in these devices the β-agonist or steroid drug is formulated as a dry powder without a propellant (i.e. they are free of CFCs). Inspiratory airflow releases the powder from the device so that they are **breath actuated**, and this reduces the problem of coordination of inspiration and inhaler actuation. The percentage of the drug delivered to the lower airways with some of these devices may be about twice that

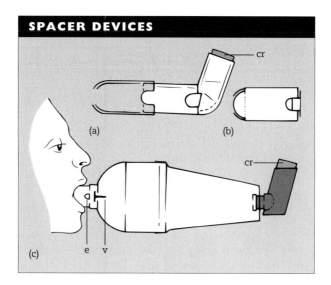

SPACER DEVICES

Fig. 11.9 Spacer devices for use with metered dose inhalers. (a) The Spacer-inhaler (Astra) is convenient and collapsible (b) and allows the patient to inhale after discharge of the aerosol; (c) the Nebuhaler (Astra) is a large-volumed device, designed to allow even freer dispersal of the discharged material so that a high proportion of it forms particles small enough to be inhaled. It also allows large doses of aerosol to be inhaled relatively efficiently (see text). cr, canister of pressurized aerosol; v, valve which closes on expiration; e, expiratory port.

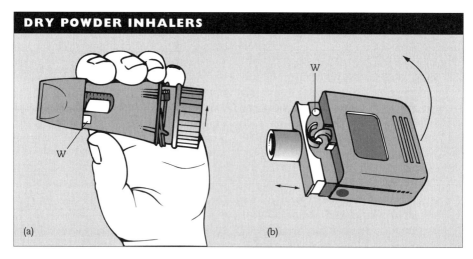

DRY POWDER INHALERS

Fig. 11.10 Dry-powder inhalers: (a) turbohaler (Astra) (b) diskhaler (Allen and Hanbury). (a) Turbohaler: the inhaler is shown with the cover removed, the mouth piece is to the left. Up to 200 doses of the powdered drug are stored in a reservoir through which the air channel passes. A dose of the dry powder is rotated into the air channel by turning the distal section (arrow). The number of doses remaining is indicated in a small window (w). (b) Diskhaler: the inhaler is shown with the mouthpiece cover removed; the mouthpiece is to the left. The individual doses are contained in sealed 'blebs' on a disk which is placed on a 'carousel' assembly inside the inhaler. With an in–out movement of the front end of the inhaler (double arrow) the disk rotates and a new bleb moves into place. The bleb is perforated before inhalation by opening the top flap (arrow). When the patient inspires, air is directed through the pierced bleb and the powder is dispersed into the airstream.

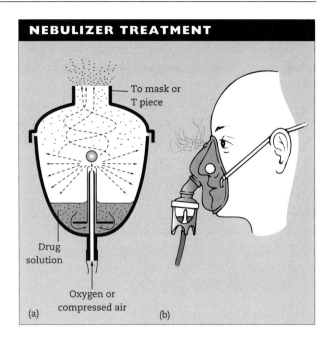

NEBULIZER TREATMENT

To mask or T piece

Drug solution

Oxygen or compressed air

(a)   (b)

Fig. 11.11 Nebulizer treatment. (a) Diagram of typical nebulization mechanism. (b) Nebulizer mask for administration of high-dose bronchodilator (see text).

delivered via a metered dose inhaler, at 20%, such that it may be possible to reduce the dose of steroids, for example, when converting from metered dose inhaler to a dry-powder device.

• *Nebulizers* (Fig. 11.11): in this form of inhaled therapy, oxygen or compressed air is directed through a narrow hole creating a local negative pressure (Venturi effect) which draws the drug solution into the air stream from a reservoir chamber. The droplets are then impacted against a small sphere, and small particles are carried as an aerosol, whereas larger particles hit the side wall of the chamber and fall back into the reservoir solution. The aerosol is administered by mask, or via a mouthpiece. Nebulizers are a convenient **means of giving high doses of bronchodilator drugs in acute attacks of asthma** where coordination of inhaler administration may be difficult in a distressed patient. They may also be used for delivering inhaled steroids (e.g. budesonide) in very young children although it is important to realize that properly used dry-powder devices, e.g. turbohaler, or metered dose inhalers and spacer devices deliver a greater percentage of the administered dose to the lower airway and

are therefore the devices of choice for routine long-term treatment. The danger of patients having machines at home for administration of bronchodilators lies in the fact that they may over-rely on the temporary alleviation of symptoms by nebulized bronchodilators to the detriment of regular anti-inflammatory therapy, and they may delay seeking urgent medical advice during acute severe asthma attacks.

Acute severe asthma

Some patients with brittle asthma are particularly susceptible to recurrent sudden attacks of severe asthma but any patient with asthma may develop an acute attack under certain circumstances (e.g. viral infection, allergen exposure). It is crucial that all patients with asthma know how to recognize the features of a severe attack and know what action to take. Each year in the UK there are about 2000 deaths certified as being due to asthma. Most of the people who die of acute asthma do so because the severity of the attack was underestimated.

The British Thoracic Society guidelines (see Further reading) therefore emphasize the importance of monitoring peak flow measurements during an attack and recognizing the features of severe asthma.

Clinical features

- Too breathless to complete sentences in one breath.
- Respiratory rate ≥ 25 breaths/min.
- Heart rate ≥ 110 beats/min.
- Peak expiratory flow $\leq 50\%$ of predicted normal or best.

Life-threatening features

- Peak expiratory flow $< 33\%$ of predicted normal or best.
- A silent chest, cyanosis, or feeble respiratory effort.
- Bradycardia or hypotension.
- Exhaustion, confusion or coma.
- Severe hypoxaemia ($Po_2 < 8$ kPa (60 mmHg)).
- Normal (5–6 kPa (38–60 mmHg)) or high Pco_2.

Immediate management

- *Oxygen*: the highest concentration available should be used. Masks delivering 24 or 28% are not appropriate.
- *High-dose nebulized β-agonist*, e.g. salbutamol 5 mg or terbutaline 10 mg. This may be repeated after 15–30 minutes if the patient's condition is not improving. Multiple doses from an inhaler should be given with a spacer device if a nebulizer is not available.
- *High-dose systemic steroid*, e.g. prednisolone 30–60 mg orally, or hydrocortisone 200 mg IV, or both, immediately.

If life threatening features are present add the following.

- *Nebulized ipratropium*: add ipratropium 0.5 mg to the nebulized β-agonist.
- *Intravenous bronchodilators*: consider adding intravenous aminophylline 250 mg IV over 20 minutes, or salbutamol or terbutaline (250 μg over 10 minutes). Do not give bolus aminophylline to patients already taking oral theophyllines.

Investigations

Arterial blood gases; urea and electrolyte concentrations; electrocardiogram in older patients; chest X-ray.

Monitoring treatment

Continued vigilance is required. The patient's condition may deteriorate some hours after an initial improvement (e.g. during the night afterwards). Measure and record peak expiratory flow 15–30 minutes after starting treatment and thereafter according to the response (at least 4 times daily measurements). Monitor respiratory rate, pulse, patient's general condition and oxygen saturation frequently. Nursing staff should be asked to call the doctor if there is a deterioration in these signs, and elective transfer of the patient to an intensive therapy unit (ITU) may be advisable so that their condition can be monitored more closely. Intermittent positive pressure ventilation is only rarely necessary but is used when the patient shows signs of exhaustion (e.g. rising Pco_2), failure to maintain oxygenation, or deterioration in vital signs.

Management during recovery in hospital and following discharge

The opportunity should be taken to improve the patient's understanding of asthma and its management, and to provide written guidance on future management. Ways of improving the patient's response to worsening asthma should be identified. Most crises resulting in hospital admission are probably preventable. The importance of peak flow measurement in determining treatment changes should be explained. Possible precipitating factors should be identified.

Patients should not normally be discharged until symptoms have resolved and lung function has stabilized or returned to normal or best levels. Nebulized bronchodilator drugs should be changed to standard inhalers 24–48 hours before discharge. Inhaler technique should be checked and performance recorded. If necessary, alternative inhaler devices should be used.

Further reading

Bascom R, Bromberg PA, Costa DL *et al.* Health effects of outdoor air pollution. *Am J Respir Crit Care Med* 1996; **153**: 477–98.

British Thoracic Society. Guidelines on the management of asthma. *Thorax* 1993; **48** (suppl. 2); Review and position statement *Thorax* 1997; **52** (suppl. 1).

Hendrick DJ. Asthma: epidemics and epidemiology. *Thorax* 1989; **44**: 609–13.

Rees J, Price J. *ABC of Asthma*. London: BMJ Publishing Group, 1996.

Tattersfield AE, Sears MR, Holgate ST *et al.* Asthma. *Lancet* 1997; **350** (suppl. II): 1–27.

CHAPTER 12

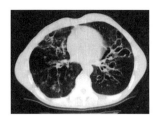

Chronic Obstructive Pulmonary Disease

Introduction

Chronic obstructive pulmonary disease (COPD) is caused mainly by smoking and its prevalence and mortality reflect the smoking history of the population. Worldwide, COPD causes about 3 million deaths each year. In the UK about 30 000 persons die and about 30 million working days are lost each year as a result of COPD.

Definitions (Table 12.1)

Chronic obstructive pulmonary disease
COPD is defined as a disease state characterized by the presence of **airflow obstruction** due to **chronic bronchitis** or **emphysema**: the airflow obstruction is generally progressive, may be accompanied by airway hyperreactivity, and may be partially reversible.

Although there is some overlap in the features of COPD and asthma, they are separate disorders with different aetiologies, pathologies, natural history and responses to treatment. In asthma, airway inflammation and hyperreactivity are the key factors giving rise to bronchial muscle contraction and airways obstruction. In COPD, structural changes arising from alveolar destruction by emphysema result in a loss of elastic recoil and a loss of outward traction on the small airways such that they collapse on expiration contributing to the airways obstruction, air trapping and hyperinflation (Figs 12.1, 12.2).

Chronic bronchitis
Chronic bronchitis is a hypersecretory disorder defined as the presence of **cough productive of sputum on most days for at least 3 months of 2 successive years** in a patient in whom other causes of a chronic cough have been excluded (e.g. tuberculosis, bronchiectasis). The diagnosis is made on the basis of symptoms. The airways of patients with chronic bronchitis show mucous gland hypertrophy and an increased number of goblet cells. The mucous gland hypertrophy may be quantified pathologically by the Reid index which is the ratio of the thickness of the mucous gland layer in the bronchial wall to the total wall thickness. Although chronic bronchitis and obstructive lung disease result from inhaling cigarette smoke they do not show a clear relationship to each other and are distinct components of the spectrum of chronic obstructive pulmonary disease. Mucus hypersecretion is mainly due to changes in the central airways whereas progressive airways obstruction arises principally from damage to the peripheral airways and alveoli.

Airways obstruction
Airways obstruction is an increased resistance

COPD

Term	Definition	Diagnosis
Chronic bronchitis	Cough and sputum for 3 months of 2 successive years	Symptoms
Airways obstruction	Diffuse airway narrowing with increased resistance to airflow	↓FEV_1/VC ↓PEF
Asthma	Reversible airways obstruction with airway inflammation and hyperresponsiveness	Bronchodilator and steroid response
Emphysema	Dilatation of the terminal airspaces with destruction of alveoli	Pathology CT scan ↓K_{CO}, ↓$T_{L}CO$
Respiratory failure	Failure to maintain oxygenation	↓Po_2 ↓O_2 sat
Cor pulmonale	Right heart hypertrophy and failure due to chronic lung disease	Oedema ↑JVP ECG ECHO

CT, computed tomography; ECG, electrocardiogram; ECHO, echocardiography; FEV_1, forced expiratory volume in 1 second; JVP, jugular vein pulse; PEF, peak expiratory flow; VC, vital capacity.

Table 12.1 Chronic obstructive pulmonary disease (COPD).

to airflow caused by diffuse airways narrowing. The term denotes a disturbance of physiology as manifest by a **reduced peak expiratory flow, forced expiratory volume in 1 second (FEV_1)** and **FEV_1/vital capacity (VC) ratio**. The diagnosis is based upon lung function tests. A number of factors contribute to airways obstruction in COPD. Loss of elastic recoil from destruction of alveoli by emphysema is an important factor in producing airway collapse. Airway inflammation is also present and provokes bronchoconstriction which is partly reversible by bronchodilator medication. Accumulation of mucous secretions and superimposed infections may aggravate airways obstruction.

The **degree of reversibility** of the airways obstruction is assessed by measuring the response to bronchodilator and corticosteroid drugs, and this varies considerably with some patients having a significant reversible component to their disease whereas others have predominantly fixed airways obstruction. The

severity of the airways obstruction may be arbitrarily graded according to the FEV_1 value: mild 60–79% of predicted, moderate 40–59% of predicted, severe < 40% of predicted.

Emphysema

Emphysema is defined in terms of its pathological features which consist of **dilatation of the terminal air spaces of the lung distal to the terminal bronchiole with destruction of their walls**. Physiologically emphysema is characterized by a reduction in the transfer factor for carbon monoxide and transfer coefficient. High-resolution computed tomography (CT) scans can demonstrate the parenchymal lung destruction of emphysema. Two main patterns of emphysema are recognized (Fig. 12.1): **centriacinar** (centrilobular) emphysema involves damage around the respiratory bronchioles with preservation of the more distal alveolar ducts and alveoli. Characteristically it affects the upper lobes and upper parts of the lower lobes of the lung. **Panaci-

EMPHYSEMA

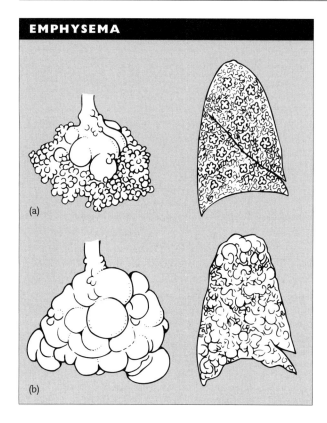

Fig. 12.1 Emphysema. Diagrammatic view of lobule and whole lung section in (a) centrilobular and (b) panacinar emphysema.

LOSS OF ELASTIC RECOIL

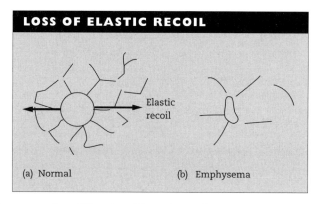

Fig. 12.2 Emphysema consists of dilatation of the terminal air spaces of the lungs, distal to the terminal bronchiole with destruction of their walls. Small peripheral airways lack cartilage and depend on the support of the surrounding alveoli to maintain their patency (a). Alveolar destruction in emphysema results in a loss of elastic recoil and a loss of outward traction on the small airways such that they collapse on expiration contributing to the airways obstruction (b).

nar (panlobular) emphysema results in distension and destruction of the whole of the acinus, and particularly affects the lower half of the lungs. Although both types of emphysema are related to smoking and may be present together, it is possible that they may arise by different mechanisms and give rise to different patterns of impairment of lung function. Panacinar emphysema is the characteristic feature of patients with α_1-anti-trypsin enzyme deficiency.

Aetiology

Tobacco smoking is the main cause of COPD such that many doctors favour the use of a simple, direct term such as 'smoker's lung' which gives a clear message to the patient about the cause of the disease and the need for smoking cessation. The total dose of tobacco inhaled is important and depends on factors such as age of starting smoking, depth of inhalation and total number of cigarettes smoked (one 'pack year' is defined as the equivalent of 20 cigarettes per day for 1 year).

Although nearly all patients with COPD have smoked heavily, only about 20% of smokers develop COPD, suggesting that additional factors such as genetic susceptibility or other environmental influences play a role. There is a higher prevalence of COPD in men than in women, in patients of lower socio-economic status and in urban rather than rural areas. The prevalence and mortality rates for COPD are higher in the north and west of England than in the south-east. Many of these geographical and demographic differences simply reflect differences in cigarette smoking habit.

There is strong evidence that COPD may be aggravated by air pollution but the role of pollution in the aetiology of COPD appears to be small when compared with that of cigarette smoking. Many dusty occupations are associated with the development of chronic bronchitis, and various forms of obstructive airways disease are associated with occupational environments, e.g. byssinosis in cotton workers, asthma in paint sprayers, obstructive airways disease in farmers (see Chapter 15). However, the contribution of occupation to the development of COPD is small when compared to the dominant effect of cigarette smoking. Nonetheless, exposure to coal dust, cotton dust and grain may be associated with an increased risk for developing COPD.

A variety of factors in early childhood have an important influence on the development of obstructive airways disease in adulthood by determining the maximum lung function achieved in adolescence and possibly also the subsequent rate of decline in lung function. Such factors include passive exposure to cigarette smoke either transplacentally in utero or environmentally in the home. Childhood respiratory illnesses including respiratory tract infections are also important. Some studies suggest that the presence of airway responsiveness predicts an accelerated rate of decline in lung function in smokers. Family and twin studies suggest that genetic factors contribute to the differences between individuals in their susceptibility to developing COPD if they smoke, but these factors are poorly defined except in the case of the inherited deficiency of anti-protease enzymes. It is thought that emphysema develops as a consequence of destruction of lung tissue by proteolytic digestion resulting from an imbalance between proteases and anti-proteases and between oxidants and anti-oxidants. Genetic deficiency of the principal anti-protease, α_1-anti-trypsin, is associated with the development of severe emphysema at a young age. α_1-anti-trypsin deficiency accounts for fewer than 1% of all cases of COPD but it is possible that other unidentified proteases may be important.

Clinical features and progression

COPD has a wide spectrum of severity.

Chronic **cough** and **sputum** production are the clinical manifestations of the mucus hypersecretion of chronic bronchitis which affects about 15% of men and 5% of women in the UK. **Infective exacerbations** of bronchitis are common and are characterized by an increased cough with purulent sputum. Non-typable unencapsulated strains of *Haemophilus influenzae* often colonize the normal upper respiratory tract. In chronic bronchitis disruption of the mucociliary defence mechanism facilitates spread of infection to the bronchial tree, where infection may provoke inflammation and a self-perpetuating vicious circle of inflammation and infection, further compromising pulmonary clearance mechanisms and aggravating airways obstruction. Many exacerbations of chronic bronchitis are associated with infection with respiratory viruses, e.g. influenza A, but other organisms implicated include *Haemophilus influenzae, Streptococcus pneumoniae, Moraxella catarrhalis* and sometimes

'atypical organisms' such as *Chlamydia pneumoniae*. Extension of infection into the lung parenchyma gives rise to **bronchopneumonia** (see Chapter 6).

The characteristic feature of airways obstruction and emphysema is gradually progressive **breathlessness** sometimes associated with wheeze. Because of the large pulmonary reserve, patients with a sedentary lifestyle often do not notice breathlessness until a great deal of lung function has been permanently lost. Figure 12.3 illustrates the insidious progressive way in which lung function is lost in COPD and shows the crucial importance of smoking cessation in slowing the rate of decline in FEV_1. Not all patients with chronic bronchitis develop airways obstruction since these are separate, although overlapping, outcomes of smoking-related lung damage. Measurement of FEV_1 and forced vital capacity (FVC) by spirometry is essential in diagnosing airways obstruction, in monitoring the pro-

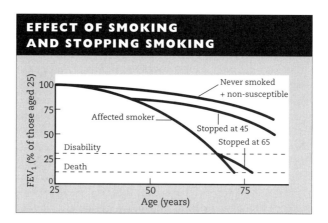

Fig. 12.3 Change in forced expiratory volume in 1 second (FEV_1) with age: effect of smoking and stopping smoking. Result of a long-term follow-up study of workers in London (an important image for doctors (and smoking patients)). Several points are illustrated: (1) non-smokers show a small progressive decline in function with age; (2) by the time disability is noted, ventilatory function is seriously reduced to about one-third of predicted normal values; (3) many smokers are unaffected by smoking and show the same decline as non-smokers; (4) some smokers are affected and show a steeper decline; (5) those affected by smoking can be detected by measurement of FEV_1 many years before they become disabled, because they will already tend to show impairment; (6) stopping smoking is not accompanied by recovery although deterioration slows to about the rate shown by non-smokers of the same age; (7) stopping smoking carries more benefit if it occurs before the development of disability; (8) continued smoking by affected smokers is associated with continued accelerated decline in function. (From Fletcher & Peto, 1977.)

gression of the disease and in assessing the response to treatment. In patients with established airways obstruction, symptoms are often aggravated by exposure to cigarette smoke, cold air, fog, atmospheric pollution and respiratory tract infections. There is generally a **gradual progression of disability** over a period of 10–40 years. This is associated with increasing absence from work, gradual limitation of exercise tolerance and a reduced range of activities. With time, **acute exacerbations** become more alarming and are accompanied by breathlessness at rest and difficulty in expectorating sputum. Admission to hospital is often required during these episodes.

As lung function deteriorates it is important to monitor oxygen levels by oximetry or arterial blood gas analysis because the symptoms of **respiratory failure** are non-specific, consisting of lethargy, tiredness, loss of energy and general malaise. Hypercapnia may cause headaches particularly on awakening in the mornings. **Cor pulmonale** is a term used to denote right ventricular hypertrophy and right heart failure secondary to chronic lung disease. The clinical features of right heart failure consist of peripheral oedema, elevation of the jugular venous pressure and hepatomegaly sometimes associated with a palpable right ventricular heave and tricuspid regurgitation.

Two main clinical patterns of disturbance may be discerned in patients with advanced COPD, which differ mainly in the extent to which ventilatory drive is preserved in the face of increasing airways obstruction: **'pink puffers'** and **'blue bloaters'** (Fig. 12.4). These

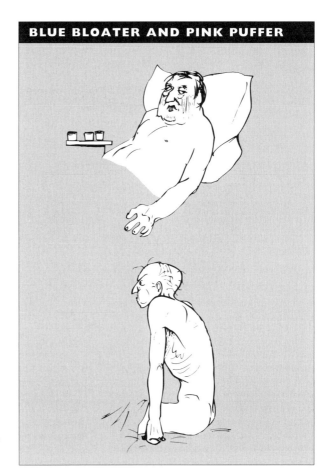

BLUE BLOATER AND PINK PUFFER

Fig. 12.4 'Blue bloater' (above) and 'pink puffer' (below). (Original drawings reproduced by kind permission of Dr R.A.L. Brewis. From *Lecture Notes on Respiratory Disease*, 1st edn.)

represent two extremes of a spectrum and most patients do not fit either pattern completely, but have some features of both. 'Pink puffers' have well-preserved ventilatory drive even in the presence of severe airways obstruction. Dyspnoea is usually intense but blood gases are often maintained in the normal range at rest until the terminal stages of the disease. 'Blue bloaters' have poor ventilatory drive and easily drift into respiratory failure with hypercapnia, hypoxaemia and right heart failure, particularly during exacerbations.

Investigations

Lung function tests

Spirometry is more accurate than peak expiratory flow measurement in assessing and monitoring the degree of airways obstruction in COPD. **Total lung capacity** and **residual volume** are often elevated signifying hyperinflation and air trapping. **Transfer** factor for carbon monoxide and **transfer coefficient** are typically reduced in emphysema.

Arterial blood gases

Oximetry is useful in measuring oxygen saturation non-invasively but a sample of **arterial blood** is necessary to assess Po_2 and Pco_2 levels.

Radiology (Fig. 12.5)

The **chest X-ray** typically shows hyperinflation of the chest with flattened low hemidiaphragms, an increased retrosternal airspace and a long narrow cardiac shadow. The chest X-ray is also an important investigation in excluding additional diagnoses, e.g. lung cancer and in detecting complications of COPD, e.g. pneumothorax, bronchopneumonia. **High-resolution CT scans** can demonstrate the extent of emphysema and the presence of bullae but are not required for the routine care of patients with COPD.

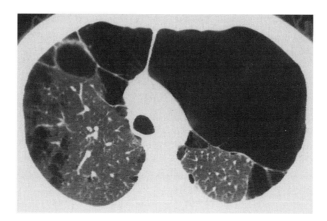

Fig. 12.5 This 42-year-old man had smoked 20 cigarettes a day since the age of 14. He presented with a 5-year history of progressive breathlessness and could walk only 100 metres. He had severe airways obstruction with a forced expiratory volume in 1 second (FEV_1) of 0.5 litres, and transfer factor for carbon monoxide and transfer coefficient were reduced to 30% of the predicted values. High-resolution computed tomography shows extensive emphysematous bullae with dilated distal airspaces, cysts and destruction of alveolar architetcture. α_1-antitrypsin levels were unrecordable. His condition continued to deteriorate and showed no response to bronchodilator medication or prednisolone. At the time of writing he was being considered for lung transplantation.

Sputum microbiology

Antibiotics are often prescribed empirically during exacerbations of COPD based upon a knowledge of the likely organisms. **Sputum culture** may be useful in confirming what organisms are present and in detecting resistance to antibiotics.

General tests

Some patients with chronic hypoxaemia develop polycythaemia with elevated **haemoglobin** levels. **White-cell count** may be elevated during infective exacerbations particularly if infection is not confined to the bronchi but has spread to the lung parenchyma as bronchopneumonia. It is important to assess for any **electrolyte** disturbance in patients with acute exacerbations requiring nebulized bronchodilator drugs. Patients with cor pulmonale may show features of right ventricular hypertrophy (right axis deviation, dominant R wave in V_1) on **electrocardiography (ECG)** and a dilated hypertrophied ventricle with tricuspid regurgitation on **echocardiography**.

Management

Management of COPD involves smoking cessation to slow the rate of decline of lung function, judicious use of drug treatments to optimize clinical status, rehabilitation and support to improve quality of life, and oxygen therapy to correct hypoxaemia when present.

Stopping smoking

It is estimated that 120 000 people die each year in the UK from smoking. Tackling an epidemic of this size requires action by all levels of society. Measures designed to discourage smoking among the young are particularly important in the primary prevention of smoking-related diseases. These include promotion of the **anti-smoking message, education** about the adverse effects of smoking, **restricting use** of tobacco in public places (e.g. in restaurants, on public transport) and in the work place, and **curtailing advertising**

of smoking by the tobacco industry. Although smoking rates are declining in the USA and Europe they are increasing in developing countries so that the epidemic of smoking-related mortality and morbidity which has dominated health trends in the Western world in the 20th century may be repeated in the developing world in the next century. There is an important role for all health-care professionals in providing leadership and example in creating a tobacco-free society. Many long-term smokers are introduced to the habit as teenagers when they are vulnerable to cigarette advertising and when smoking may be seen as a symbol of 'forbidden' adult behaviour. Counteracting such rebellious youth culture is difficult but involves the promotion of a **positive image of a healthy lifestyle** and emphasizing the **unattractiveness of the smoker** whose clothes, hands and breath reek of tobacco. Outright prohibition of smoking is not likely to be feasible or successful but the example of parents, teachers, sports people and society in general is crucial.

Patients with COPD who continue to smoke show an accelerated rate of decline in lung function. Conversely stopping smoking slows the rate of decline to the same rate as in non-smokers. All patients with COPD should be made aware of this and urged to stop smoking. When speaking to patients, the use of a direct term such as **'smoker's lung'** rather than COPD may be useful. Smoking cessation is notoriously difficult and the patient requires **support** and **encouragement**. It is important that other members of the **patient's family** adopt a positive supporting attitude and also stop smoking. It may be helpful for the patient to initially **monitor his or her smoking behaviour:** How much? When? Why? In what circumstances? A goal is then set including a **target date for quitting**. The patient needs to avoid situations previously associated with smoking and to substitute other activities.

A positive attitude to smoking cessation fosters a greater belief in the patient's personal control of life and health. The highest success rates in stopping smoking are seen in patients who have suffered a myocardial infarction or a major respiratory illness when powerful advice about risk to life is given. Some patients experience **withdrawal symptoms** such as irritability, restlessness and sleep disturbance which may last up to 4 weeks, and **nicotine chewing gum** or transdermal **nicotine patches** may sometimes be helpful. When cessation has been achieved it is important to continue support and encouragement to **prevent relapse**. Exhaled carbon monoxide levels may be used to validate smoking cessation with values greater than about 10 p.p.m. suggesting on-going smoking.

Drug treatment (see also Chapter 11)
Bronchodilators
Most patients with COPD show some response to bronchodilator drugs although this is less than is seen in patients with asthma. Nonetheless, small improvements in airways obstruction can produce important benefits in terms of relief of breathlessness, reduction in the degree of air trapping and improved exercise capacity. β_2-**agonists** such as salbutamol and terbutaline relax bronchial smooth muscle by stimulation of β-adrenoceptors. **Long-acting β-agonists** such as salmeterol and formoterol give more prolonged relief of symptoms and may be particularly useful in relieving nocturnal symptoms. **Anticholinergic** drugs such as ipratropium and oxitropium produce bronchodilatation by blocking the bronchoconstrictor effect of vagal nerve stimulation of bronchial smooth muscle. **Methylxanthines** such as aminophylline and theophyllines have a number of effects including cyclic adenosine monophosphate (AMP) stimulation of β-adrenoceptors by inhibiting the metabolism of cyclic AMP by the enzyme phosphodiesterase.

Corticosteroids
About 20–30% of patients with COPD improve if given oral steroid therapy. In order to detect this subgroup of patients and to determine the degree of steroid reversibility of their disease patients with significant airways obstruction and symptoms should be given a formal **trial of prednisolone 30 mg/day for about 14 days** during a stable phase. Patients with a significant response to steroids should be treated with long-term inhaled corticosteroids. Patients who fail to respond to this formal trial of oral prednisolone are not usually treated with inhaled steroids. However, there is considerable interest in whether inhaled steroids have a role in ameliorating the rate of decline in lung function in patients with COPD, and a number of studies including EUROSCOP (European Study of Chronic Obstructive Pulmonary Disease) and ISOLDE (International Study of Obstructive Lung Disease) are addressing this question.

Serial spirometry measurements are useful in assessing the response to treatment. Drug therapy is often deployed in a stepwise fashion depending on the severity of the disease and level of symptoms. Even a slight improvement in airways obstruction may have significant benefits in relieving symptoms in a disabled patient. However, even after optimal use of drug treatments many patients are left with residual disability, and continuing intensification of drug treatment is unlikely to be helpful since much of the lung function deficit is due to reduced elastic recoil and increased compliance of emphysema, and is not amenable to bronchodilator or corticosteroid medication (the terms **'fixed'** or **'irreversible' airways obstruction** are sometimes used to refer to this component of the disease).

Antibiotics
In some cases exacerbations of COPD are associated with infections with viruses or with bacteria such as *Haemophilus influenzae*, *Streptococcus pneumoniae* or *Moraxella catarrhalis*. Although **amoxycillin** has a reasonably good spectrum of activity against many of these organisms 15–20% of *Haemophilus influenzae* and many strains of *Moraxella catarrhalis* are resistant to **amoxycillin** so that other anti-

biotics such as **co-amoxiclav** (amoxycillin and clavulanic acid), **trimethoprim**, **cipro-floxacin**, **tetracycline** or **clarithromycin** may be needed. Sputum microbiology is useful in guiding antibiotic therapy. In many cases exacerbations of COPD seem to arise as a result of spontaneous deterioration in the disease process or are provoked by non-infectious events such as air pollution, smoking or adverse weather conditions. It may be difficult to judge the importance of using an antibiotic as one element alongside use of bron-chodilators, steroids, oxygen and sputum clear-ance techniques in exacerbations of COPD (Table 12.2). There is evidence of the beneficial effect of antibiotics in hastening the rate of recovery **in severe exacerbations** of COPD associated with increasing cough, sputum pro-duction and dyspnoea but there is no definite evidence of the benefit of antibiotics in mild exacerbations. **Long-term prophylactic antibiotics** are sometimes given to patients experiencing frequent exacerbations but there is a risk of promoting infection with resistant organisms. **Influenza vaccine** is recom-mended for patients with COPD, and pneumo-coccal vaccine may be useful.

Rehabilitation and support

Pulmonary rehabilitation involves a compre-hensive multi-disciplinary approach to **allevia-tion of symptoms** and to **optimizing the daily functioning** and **quality of life** of patients suffering from impairment and disabil-ity due to chronic respiratory disease. The success of a rehabilitation programme depends on the enthusiasm of the medical team and the motivation of the patient and his or her family. The programme should be tailored to the indi-vidual patient's needs but the principal ele-

---

TREATMENT OF SEVERE EXACERBATIONS OF COPD

Tests
Chest X-ray, oximetry, arterial blood gases, peak flow, electrocardiography, sputum culture, blood count, urea, electrolytes

Treatment
- Bronchodilators, e.g. nebulized **salbutamol** 2.5–5 mg and **ipratropium** 250–500 µg; repeat as needed and continue 4–6 hourly. If deteriorating consider aminophylline infusion

- Steroids: **hydrocortisone** 100 mg IV bolus and **prednisolone** 30 mg orally

- Oxygen: aim for O_2 sat. >90% without provoking hypercapnia and acidaemia using **controlled oxygen therapy** (e.g. 24% Venturi mask) as necessary

- Respiratory stimulants: if P_{CO_2} is rising and pH falling add **doxapram** IV infusion (e.g. 4 mg/min × 15 min, 3 mg/min × 15 min, then 2 mg/min maintenance)

- Antibiotics, e.g. amoxycillin 500 mg t.i.d. orally or IV. Check previous sputum microbiology and consider ciprofloxacin, clarithromycin, co-amoxiclav if needed

- Physiotherapy: may help **clear secretions.** The patient should be nursed sitting upright

- Additional treatments: consider need for diuretics e.g. **frusemide** 40 mg IV if in cardiac failure; or venesection if severe polycythaemia (e.g. PCV >58%)

- Mechanical ventilation in intensive therapy unit: should be considered if the patient is tiring with rising P_{CO_2} and falling pH

PCV, packed cell volume.

Table 12.2 Treatment of severe exacerbations of chronic obstructive pulmonary disease (COPD).

ments of a programme include the following (Fig. 12.6).

• *Smoking cessation*: advice, encouragement and support in achieving and maintaining smoking cessation.

• *Optimizing drug treatment*: assessing reversibility to steroid and bronchodilator drugs, optimizing treatment and instituting long-term oxygen therapy where indicated.

• *Education* of the patient and family about the nature and cause of the disease with the aim of improving the patient's ability to cope with disability and to comply with medication, oxygen therapy and smoking cessation.

• *Exercise training*: breathless patients often reduce their level of exercise and lose general fitness and muscle mass which cause a vicious

cycle of deteriorating exercise capacity. Exercise training (e.g. walking, cycling) can counteract muscle atrophy and improve fitness. Improvement in lower limb function may help walking, and arm training improves performance of day-to-day tasks such as lifting, dressing, washing and brushing hair, for example.

• *Breathing control techniques* involve pursed lip breathing, slower deeper respirations and better coordination of breathing patterns. Physiotherapy techniques such as postural drainage, chest percussion and forced expiratory techniques may be useful in patients who have difficulty expectorating secretions.

• *Psychosocial support*: patients with advanced disability may have difficulty in performing daily tasks such as climbing stairs, shopping and washing, and may benefit from help from community nurses and from home aids such as stairlifts and bath aids. Depression and social isolation are common and can be helped by psychological support focusing on restoring coping skills. Patient self-help groups may be useful. Assessment by a social worker allows the patient to obtain appropriate allowances,

Fig. 12.6 The chronic obstructive pulmonary disease (COPD) escalator. Summary of the principal components of a management plan for COPD. Note that, as disease severity increases, symptoms and signs become more obvious whilst the number of treatments used rises. (Reproduced with permission from *Thorax*. British Thoracic Society guidelines on the management of COPD. *Thorax* 1997; **52** (Suppl. 5).)

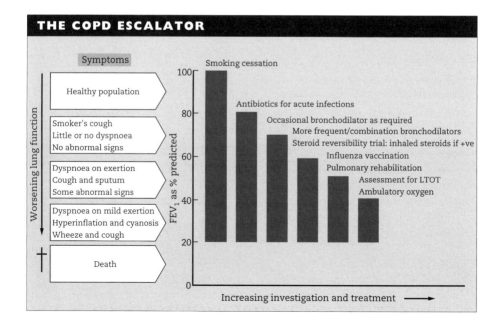

such as disability or mobility allowances, from government agencies.

• *Nutrition*: obesity is common and weight reduction can greatly improve exercise capacity. Some patients, however, suffer from cachexia and loss of muscle mass as energy expenditure is often increased by the work of breathing. Nutritional supplements may then be required.

In measuring the outcome of pulmonary rehabilitation it is important to include, not only measurements of lung function and oxygenation, but also exercise capacity, quality of life and dyspnoea scores and assessment of activities of daily living.

Surgery

A small number of patients with COPD may benefit from surgery. **Lung transplantation** is an option particularly for patients with emphysema due to α_1-anti-trypsin deficiency, although lack of donor organs severely limits the application of this procedure. **Bullectomy** may be appropriate where a large bulla is compressing surrounding viable lung. In recent years **volume reduction surgery** is being attempted in selected patients with severe disability. In emphysema, destruction of the alveoli results in a loss of elastic recoil with collapse of small airways on expiration and hyperinflation of the lungs with flattening of the diaphragm. Volume reduction surgery aims to resect functionally useless areas of lung thereby reducing the overall volume of the lungs in order to restore elastic recoil so that there is an increased outward traction on the small airways, relief of compression of normal lung and restoration of more normal diaphragmatic and thoracic contours allowing better respiratory motion during breathing. Patients whose emphysema preferentially affects the upper lobes may be the most suitable patients for this procedure.

Oxygen therapy

Oxygen delivery to the tissues of the body depends upon the inspired oxygen concentration, ventilation, gas exchange and distribution in the circulation. **Oxygen therapy** should be prescribed with due attention to the **dose** and **method of administration** and with careful **monitoring of its effects**. It is also important to optimize oxygen transport to the tissues by ensuring adequate haemoglobin level, cardiac output and tissue perfusion. Oximetry and arterial blood gas analysis are essential in initiating, monitoring and adjusting oxygen therapy.

Method of administration

An inspired concentration of 100% oxygen can only be achieved in the context of **artificial ventilation** in an intensive therapy unit (ITU) or with apparatus which provides a complete seal from the outside air and a non-return valve. High concentrations (e.g. 60–90%) can be administered via a tight-fitting face mask attached to a **reservoir bag**, although there is a potential for rebreathing of exhaled carbon dioxide. Concentrations of about 40–60% can be achieved with **simple masks in which oxygen is supplied directly to the mask space** (Fig. 12.7). The effective concentration achieved depends upon the oxygen flow and on the pattern of breathing since some air from the room is drawn into the mask diluting the oxygen concentration. **Nasal cannulae** (prongs) are the most convenient way of administering oxygen since, in contrast to masks, they are relatively unobtrusive and do not interfere with speech or eating. They are usually well tolerated and kept in place continuously so that oxygen therapy is not interrupted during sleeping or eating. The oxygen concentration administered via nasal cannulae varies not only with the oxygen flow rate but also with the patient's ventilatory rate, tidal volume and degree of mouth breathing, so that it cannot be accurately predicted and provides a relatively 'uncontrolled' form of oxygen therapy. If an accurate and constantly controlled concentration of oxygen is required then a **fixed performance Venturi mask** is necessary. Oxygen flow from a specifically designed pinhole orifice creates a local negative pressure which entrains a constant

OXYGEN ADMINISTRATION

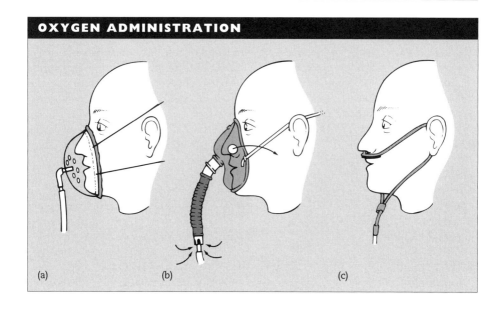

(a)   (b)   (c)

Fig. 12.7 Oxygen administration: (a) simple uncontrolled high concentration face mask with oxygen supplied directly to the mask space. (b) Fixed performance Venturi mask delivering a controlled dose of low-concentration oxygen. (c) Nasal cannulae delivering an uncontrolled level of oxygen in a convenient continuous manner.

proportion of room air through side ports at the base of the mask (small arrows, Fig. 12.7b). A selection of masks giving 24, 28 and 35% is available and the concentration delivered is dependent upon the size of the pinhole and the designs of the apertures and is relatively independent of the patient's pattern of breathing. Humidification of inspired oxygen is only needed when it is delivered directly to the trachea or at high flow rates, otherwise the oropharynx provides adequate humidification.

Acute oxygen therapy

High-concentration oxygen should be given empirically in cases of cardiac or respiratory arrest or in acute life-threatening situations (e.g. acute severe asthma). Patients with established respiratory failure who have chronically raised P_{CO_2} (type 2 respiratory failure) become unresponsive to the carbon dioxide stimulus to ventilation and rely increasingly on hypoxaemia to maintain the drive to breathe. If they are given high concentrations of oxygen they breathe less and underbreathing results in increasing hypercapnia, narcosis and ultimately respiratory depression. Uncontrolled oxygen therapy poses a risk to a subset of patients with COPD (notably 'blue bloaters' with hypercapnic (type 2) respiratory failure), although this risk has often been exaggerated and must be balanced against the threat of hypoxaemia.

Because of the shape of the oxyhaemoglobin dissociation curve there is little benefit in increasing the patient's oxygen saturation above about 90% or the P_{O_2} above about 8 kPa (60 mmHg). In treating patients with acute exacerbations of COPD, therefore, the aim of oxygen therapy is to correct hypoxaemia to a P_{O_2} >8 kPa (60 mmHg) or oxygen saturation >90% without provoking critical hypercapnia and respiratory acidosis. Very often this can be achieved by measuring oximetry with the patient breathing air and then giving controlled oxygen therapy, e.g. using a 24 or 28% fixed performance Venturi mask to achieve an oxygen saturation above 90%. Arterial blood gases are then analysed when the patient has been breathing the required amount of oxygen for about 30 minutes. If the P_{CO_2} is below 6 kPa (45 mmHg) then it is safe to transfer to nasal cannulae using oximetry to determine the flow rate required (e.g. 1–2 L/min) to maintain oxygen saturation just above 90%. If the P_{CO_2} is above 6 kPa (45 mmHg) then it is advisable to continue oxygen therapy using a fixed performance mask. If P_{CO_2} is greater than 8 kPa (60 mmHg), or rises further with a fall in pH during oxygen therapy then a respiratory stimulant such as **doxapram** may be useful in stimulating ventilation.

Judicious use of oximetry and measurement of arterial blood gases under precisely judged circumstances (e.g. when the patient has reached steady state on the required concentration of oxygen as judged by oximetry) can limit the need for repeated arterial blood sampling. It is essential to document carefully the amount of oxygen being breathed when measuring arterial gases. Avoid measuring gases immediately after the patient has received nebulized drugs using high-flow oxygen. Sometimes there is concern about using high-flow oxygen (e.g. 6–8 L/min) to nebulize bronchodilator drugs in patients with hypercapnia and occasionally air is used to nebulize these drugs. However, nebulizing drugs using air during acute exacerbations of COPD may leave the patient dangerously hypoxic and it is probably better to continue using oxygen 6–8 L/min to nebulize the drug but to limit the nebulization time strictly to 10–15 minutes so that the patient is not exposed to the risk of either hypoxia or prolonged high-concentration oxygen.

Repeat arterial gas measurements are required if the patient's condition deteriorates. A rising P_{CO_2} and a falling pH indicate progressive respiratory failure and failing ventilation requiring consideration for full endotracheal mechanical ventilation in an ITU or non-invasive intermittent positive pressure ventilation (NIPPV) via a tight-fitting nasal mask (see Chapter 19). In some cases the patient's under-lying disease has progressed to a stage where mechanical ventilation in ITU is unlikely to be successful and a palliative approach towards relief of symptoms is more appropriate than futile treatment which may merely prolong the process of dying to the distress of the patient and his or her relatives. On the other hand, ventilation may be life saving for patients who have previously had a reasonable level of respiratory function and who have potentially correctable factors contributing to the acute crisis (e.g. pneumonia, pneumothorax, etc.). It is important to seek advice early from senior medical staff and ITU staff for patients with deteriorating respiratory failure.

Long-term oxygen therapy

Patients with COPD and chronic hypoxaemia have a poor prognosis with a mortality rate of about 50% within 3 years. The clinical features of hypoxaemia are non-specific, and periodic measurement of oxygen saturation by oximetry is useful in detecting these patients. Hypoxaemia is a powerful stimulus to pulmonary artery vasoconstriction which if persistent provokes pulmonary hypertension, right ventricular hypertrophy and right heart failure (cor pulmonale). In the early 1980s two major studies, the American Nocturnal Oxygen Therapy Trial (NOTT) and the British Medical Research Council (MRC) Study, showed that the administration of oxygen for at least 15 hours daily (preferably longer) improved survival in patients with severe airflow obstruction (FEV$_1$ < 1.5 litres) and hypoxaemia (P_{O_2} < 7.3 kPa (55 mmHg)) who had peripheral oedema.

Prescribing criteria

Long-term home oxygen therapy is indicated for **non-smoking patients with severe COPD (FEV$_1$ < 1.5 litres) and persistent hypoxaemia (P_{O_2} < 7.3 kPa (55 mmHg))**. Many patients who are hypoxaemic during an exacerbation will recover over a few weeks and will not require long-term oxygen. Arterial blood gases should therefore be measured on two occasions, at least 3 weeks apart, during a stable phase before diagnosing persistent hypoxaemia. Patients with more borderline oxygen levels (7.3–8.0 kPa (55–60 mmHg)) who have elevated haematocrit or features of cor pulmonale such as oedema are also likely to benefit from long-term oxygen. The oxygen is usually given via nasal cannulae at a flow rate of about 2 L/min but the dose required and mode of administration should be decided by a hospital specialist in the context of the patient's arterial blood gas measurement.

Oxygen concentrator

Long-term home oxygen therapy is provided from an oxygen concentrator. This is an electrically powered machine which separates oxygen from the ambient air using a molecular sieve. The machine is installed in the patient's house and plastic tubing relays oxygen to points such as the bedroom and living room. Providing oxygen cylinders to the patient's home for long-term oxygen therapy is impractical and much more expensive than installation of an oxygen concentrator. The patient and family should be warned not to smoke in the presence of oxygen because of the risk of causing a fire. It is essential that the patient understands that the main aim of long-term oxygen therapy is to improve prognosis (reduce mortality rate) rather than to alleviate symptoms and that it is necessary to comply with oxygen therapy for at least 15 hours daily. The patient achieves this by using oxygen during sleep at night and whilst ordinary domestic activities are performed during the day.

Further reading

American Thoracic Society. Standards for the diagnosis and care of patients with chronic obstructive pulmonary disease. *Am J Respir Crit Care Med* 1995; **152**: S78–S120.

British Thoracic Society. Guidelines on the management of chronic obstructive pulmonary disease. *Thorax* 1997; **52** (suppl. 5).

Donner CF, Muir JF. Selection criteria and programmes for pulmonary rehabilitation in COPD patients. *Eur Respir J* 1997; **10**: 744–57.

Fletcher C, Peto R. The natural history of chronic airflow obstruction. *BMJ* 1977; **1**: 1645.

Jayanthi V, Probert CSJ, Sher KS, Mayberry JF. Smoking and prevention. *Respir Med* 1991; **85**: 179–83.

Leach RM, Bateman NT. Acute oxygen therapy. *Br J Hosp Med* 1993; **49**: 637–44.

CHAPTER 13

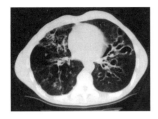

Carcinoma of the Lung

Introduction

Although largely preventable, carcinoma of the lung kills about 38 000 people each year in the UK. It is the commonest cause of cancer death in men and the second commonest cause in women, after breast cancer.

Aetiology (Table 13.1)

The epidemic spread of lung cancer in the 20th century followed about 20 years after increases in **tobacco-smoking** habits (Fig. 13.1). The commercial manufacture of cigarettes started around 1900 and smoking soon became popular amongst men. In the 1920s women adopted the habit. By the end of the 1940s about 70% of men and 40% of women smoked. By 1950 an epidemic of lung cancer had become apparent and studies, such as those of Doll and Hill in the 1950s, established the link between smoking and lung cancer. The risk of death from bronchial carcinoma increases by a factor roughly equal to the number of cigarettes smoked per day. For example, a man smoking 30 cigarettes/day has over 30 times the risk of dying from lung cancer than a man who has never smoked. On stopping smoking, excess risk is approximately halved every 5 years thereafter. Smoking has decreased in popularity such that now about

31% of men and 29% of women smoke. Reflecting these changes, lung cancer mortality rates have recently begun to decline in men and in younger women, although rates in older women are still rising. Smoking habits vary and are at their highest in the north of England and Scotland where lung cancer has overtaken breast cancer as the commonest cause of cancer death in women. Although smoking in the UK is declining, it is increasing in developing countries so that the epidemic of smoking-related mortality and morbidity which has dominated health trends in the Western world in the 20th century may be repeated in the developing world in the next century.

Breathing other people's tobacco smoke — **passive smoking** — is also a cause of lung cancer. For example, a woman who has never smoked has an estimated 24% greater risk of developing lung cancer if she lives with a smoker. The increased rate of lung cancer in **urban** compared with rural areas may simply reflect different smoking habits rather than an influence of environmental **pollution**. **Genetic factors** probably determine susceptibility to smoking. For example, the degree of induction of the aryl hydrocarbon hydroxylase enzyme system may be genetically determined and can activate hydrocarbons in cigarette smoke into carcinogens. There is an increased incidence of lung cancer in patients with **diffuse lung fibrosis** such as cryptogenic fibrosing alveolitis or scleroderma; and so-

LUNG CANCER AETIOLOGY

Tobacco smoking
Passive smoking
Genetic factors
Urban environment
Ionizing radiation (e.g. radon gas)
Asbestos exposure
Diffuse lung fibrosis (e.g. fibrosing alveolitis)
Lack of dietary fruit and vegetables

Table 13.1 Aetiology of carcinoma of the lung.

called '**scar carcinomas**' may occur in areas of focal fibrosis resulting from previous tuberculosis. Some studies suggest that a high dietary intake of fruit and vegetables containing β-carotene reduces the risk of lung cancer. Exposure to **ionizing radiation** such as from radon gas arising from the ground and building materials in some homes may be important and account for a proportion of lung cancers in non-smokers. Occupational exposure to **asbestos** is associated with an increased risk of lung cancer with an approximately linear relationship between the dose of asbestos and the occurrence of lung cancer. The interac-

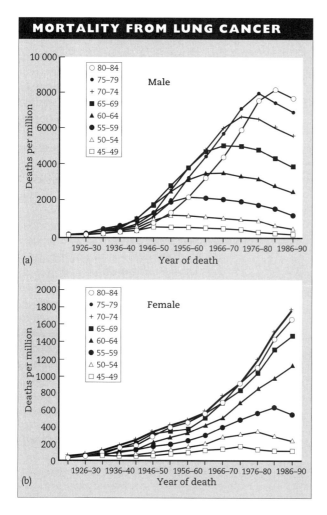

Fig. 13.1 (a) Male mortality and (b) female mortality from lung cancer by age and year of death, England and Wales, 1921–90. (Reproduced with permission from the Lung and Asthma Information Agency. From *Trends in Lung Cancer and Smoking*. Factsheet 93/1.)

tion between asbestos and smoking is multiplicative.

Pathology (Fig. 13.2)

Although the pathology of lung cancer is complex, for clinical purposes the disease is classified into two groups:
1 **small-cell carcinoma** (25% of lung cancer);
2 **non-small-cell carcinoma** (75%), comprising **squamous cell carcinoma** (45%), **adenocarcinoma** (20%) and **large-cell (undifferentiated) carcinoma** (10%).
Small-cell (oat-cell) carcinoma arises from neuroendocrine cells of the bronchial tree and its endocrine potential is sometimes manifest clinically by ectopic hormone production. This is a highly malignant cancer which grows rapidly and metastasizes early. Squamous cell carcinoma is the commonest type of lung cancer and shows the greatest tendency to cavitate. The incidence of adenocarcinomas

seems to be rising and is currently about 20%. These tumours often arise in the periphery of the lung, sometimes as 'scar carcinomas' and show the least relationship to smoking. About 10% of lung cancers do not show squamous or glandular differentiation and are classified as large cell undifferentiated carcinomas.

Diagnosis

Lung cancers arising centrally in the bronchial tree often present with **chest symptoms** (e.g. haemoptysis) whereas peripheral tumours may grow silently without causing local symptoms until late in the course of the disease (Fig. 13.3). Such tumours may be found coincidentally on a **chest X-ray** or present with non-specific **general symptoms** (e.g. weight loss), with effects of **metastases** (e.g. to brain, bone) or with non-metastatic **paraneoplastic syndromes**.

Paraneoplastic syndromes arise at sites distant from the tumour or its metastases and

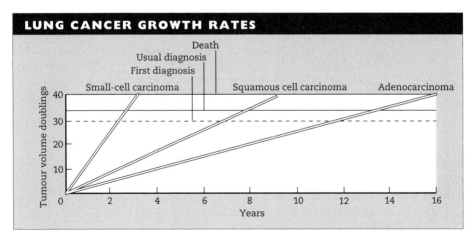

Fig. 13.2 Lung cancer growth rates. As a rough approximation, small-cell carcinomas double monthly, squamous cell carcinomas 3 monthly and some adenocarcinomas 6 monthly. A tumour typically becomes evident on a chest X-ray when it reaches about 1 cm in diameter corresponding to about 30 doubling volumes. Symptoms usually arise later than this. By 40 doublings death will

usually have occurred. Diagnosis occurs late in the course of the disease and most of the tumour's life history is subclinical. Attempts at diagnosing the subclinical phase using chest X-ray as a screening procedure make little impact on the tumour's life history and have been found to have no effect on mortality.

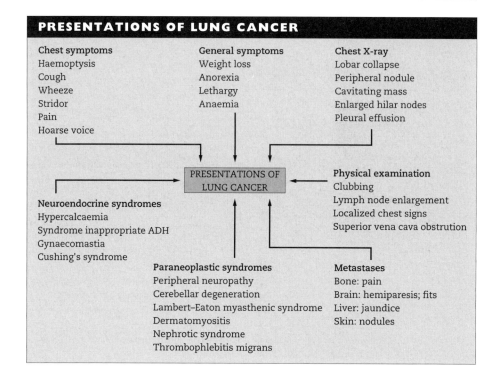

PRESENTATIONS OF LUNG CANCER

Chest symptoms
Haemoptysis
Cough
Wheeze
Stridor
Pain
Hoarse voice

General symptoms
Weight loss
Anorexia
Lethargy
Anaemia

Chest X-ray
Lobar collapse
Peripheral nodule
Cavitating mass
Enlarged hilar nodes
Pleural effusion

PRESENTATIONS OF
LUNG CANCER

Neuroendocrine syndromes
Hypercalcaemia
Syndrome inappropriate ADH
Gynaecomastia
Cushing's syndrome

Physical examination
Clubbing
Lymph node enlargement
Localized chest signs
Superior vena cava obstrution

Paraneoplastic syndromes
Peripheral neuropathy
Cerebellar degeneration
Lambert–Eaton myasthenic syndrome
Dermatomyositis
Nephrotic syndrome
Thrombophlebitis migrans

Metastases
Bone: pain
Brain: hemiparesis; fits
Liver: jaundice
Skin: nodules

Fig. 13.3 Presentations of lung cancer.

result from the production of hormones, peptides, antibodies, prostaglandins or cytokines by the tumour. The syndrome of inappropriate anti-diuretic hormone (ADH) secretion is commonest with small-cell cancer and results in a low serum sodium, potassium and urea, a serum osmolarity below 280 mosmol/l and a urine osmolarity greater than 500 mosmol/l. Treatment consists of restriction of fluid intake, and demeclocycline 600–1200 mg/day since this drug competes for ADH renal tubular binding sites. Hypercalcaemia in patients with lung cancer may be indicative of bone metastases but squamous cell carcinomas sometimes secrete a parathyroid hormone-related protein which causes non-metastatic hypercalcaemia. Clearly some patients will present primarily with chest symptoms, often against a background of pre-existing smoking-

related lung disease (e.g. chronic obstructive pulmonary disease (COPD)). Equally a diagnosis of lung cancer must be considered in patients presenting with a variety of medical problems.

Tumours in certain specific locations may cause problems by direct invasion of adjacent structures. Direct invasion of the mediastinum may cause paralysis of the **phrenic nerve**, manifest by elevation of the hemidiaphragm, or of the **recurrent laryngeal nerve**, particularly on the left side where it passes around the aortic arch to the superior mediastinum, causing vocal cord palsy with hoarseness and diminished cough reflex. Injection of Teflon into the paralysed vocal cord under general anaesthesia can improve voice quality by building up the volume of the vocal cord enabling better apposition. **Obstruction of the superior vena cava** causes venous engorgement of the upper body with facial oedema, headache, distended pulseless jugular veins and

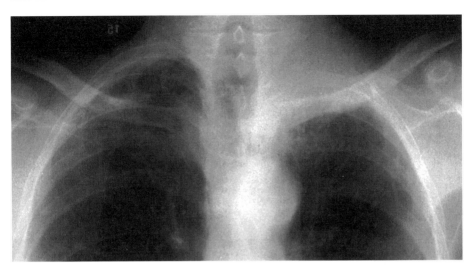

Fig. 13.4 Pancoast tumour. This 68-year-old man presented with a 3-month history of left shoulder pain. On examination he had features of a left Horner's syndrome (ptosis, meiosis, enophthalmos, anhydrosis). Chest X-ray shows a mass at the apex of the left lung eroding the first and second ribs posteriorly. Percutaneous biopsy showed squamous cell carcinoma. He was treated with palliative radiotherapy.

enlarged collateral veins over the chest and arms. These symptoms require urgent treatment by chemotherapy in the case of small-cell cancer or radiotherapy in the case of other tumours. Occasionally insertion of an expandable metallic wire stent into the strictured vein under radiological guidance is useful in relieving symptoms. A **Pancoast tumour** (Fig. 13.4) is a carcinoma situated in the superior sulcus of the lung where the subclavian artery forms a groove over the lung apex. Because of its particular anatomical location a tumour here gives rise to a characteristic syndrome: ipsilateral Horner's syndrome (ptosis, meiosis, enophthalmos, anhydrosis) due to stellate ganglion involvement; pain due to erosion of the posterior first and second ribs, and wasting of the small muscles of the hand due to brachial plexus invasion. The tumour may invade a vertebral foramen giving spinal cord compression. These tumours are notoriously difficult to detect on a chest X-ray and the cause of the patient's pain is often misdiagnosed initially.

The chest X-ray plays a pivotal role in the investigation of lung cancer, and a range of abnormalities may be apparent. A peripheral tumour may be seen as a small nodule or mass in the lung field. A cavitating mass is characteristic of squamous cell carcinoma (Fig. 4.7, p. 36). Central tumours may cause bronchial obstruction typically giving rise to atelectatic collapse of a lung or lobe of a lung (Fig. 13.5), or to pneumonic consolidation distal to the obstruction. Thus, 'loss of volume' of a lobe (atelectatic collapse) on a chest X-ray in a patient with apparent pneumonia is a sinister feature suggesting bronchial obstruction by a carcinoma. The chest X-ray may show evidence of spread of the tumour to bone (e.g. rib or

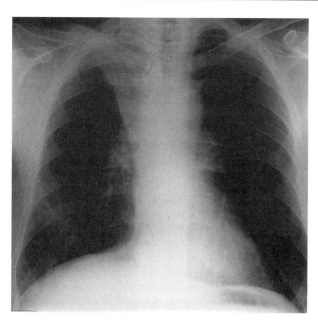

Fig. 13.5 Right upper lobe collapse. This 65-year-old smoker presented with haemoptysis. Chest X-ray shows a triangular-shaped opacity in the right upper zone indicating collapse of the right upper lobe. Bronchoscopy showed a tumour occluding the orifice to the right upper lobe and biopsy showed a large-cell undifferentiated carcinoma. Computed tomography showed that the tumour was confined to the right upper lobe without mediastinal invasion or metastases. He was treated by right upper lobectomy.

vertebral destruction), pleura (e.g. effusion), hilar or mediastinal structures.

Histological–cytological diagnosis should be obtained wherever possible. **Sputum cytology** is positive in about 40% of cases of lung cancer with the highest yield for central tumours. A series of early morning samples expectorated from deep in the chest gives the best yield. **Bronchoscopy** (Fig. 13.6) allows direct visualization and biopsy of central tumours. Peripheral tumours seen on chest X-ray may not be accessible to bronchoscopy and **percutaneous needle biopsy** of these lesions under radiological guidance is a useful technique. Small peripheral cancers need to be distinguished from rare benign tumours (e.g. hamartomas) and from granulomas resulting from previous tuberculosis, but it may be advisable to proceed to surgical resection without histological confirmation of the diagnosis if the risk of cancer is high. Diagnosis may also be achieved by obtaining material from a site of metastasis (e.g. lymph node, skin, pleural effusion).

Communicating the diagnosis

Telling a patient of the diagnosis of lung cancer is a difficult clinical skill which needs to be developed by training and experience. Patients want to talk honestly about what is happening to them and to know more about the way ahead. The patient's awareness of the diagnosis often emerges over a number of consultations and the time that elapses between initial suspicion of tumour and histological confirmation of the diagnosis is often useful in allowing the patient an opportunity to come to terms with the situation. When discussing the diagnosis it is essential to allow adequate time for questions, to ensure privacy during the interview,

BRONCHOSCOPY

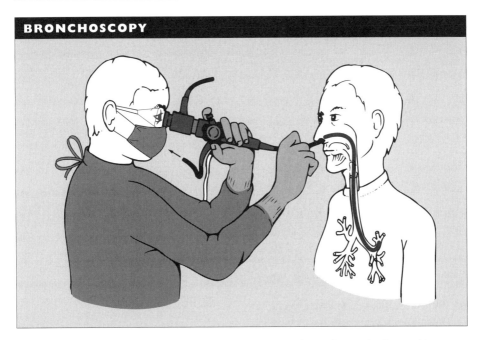

Fig. 13.6 Bronchoscopy. Flexible fibreoptic bronchoscopy is usually performed as an outpatient procedure under sedation (e.g. midazolam) and topical anaesthesia (e.g. lignocaine to vocal cords and airways). The bronchoscope is usually passed transnasally into the oropharynx, through the vocal cords into the trachea and bronchi to the subsegmental level. The bronchial tree is illuminated by light transmitted from a light source to the tip of the bronchoscope and the image is transmitted to the eyepiece or displayed on a screen. About two-thirds of lung cancers are visible through the bronchoscope, and therefore bronchoscopy is a key investigation for lung cancer or haemoptysis. A biopsy forceps or cytology brush may be passed through a channel to obtain samples from a tumour, and secretions and saline washings can be aspirated for cytology or microbiology tests. Bronchoscopy is a very safe procedure but is contraindicated in patients with uncontrolled angina or recent myocardial infarction. Sedation should be avoided or used with particular caution in patients with respiratory depression. Pulse oximetry is used to monitor oxygen saturation and supplemental oxygen is given. The scope is carefully cleaned with detergent and immersed in glutaraldehyde to prevent transmission of infection to patients. It is recommended that the bronchoscopist and nurse should wear masks, goggles and gowns to prevent contracting infections (e.g. tuberculosis) from the patient by aerosols generated by coughing.

to encourage a relative or friend to accompany the patient for support and to have further counselling available for the patient from skilled nurses. Some patients may find written information about lung cancer and its treatment useful.

Inevitably patients will experience emotions such as shock, anger and denial and the doctor must work through these emotions with the patient. It is useful to be able to bring the interview to a conclusion on a more positive note by discussing a management plan. Many patients will initially be too shocked to understand the information given and it is often useful to arrange a further interview either with the hospital doctor, nurse or general practitioner to answer the patient's questions. Rapid communication between all members of the medical team is crucial in these circumstances.

Treatment (Fig. 13.7)

Treatment depends mainly on the histological cell type and the stage of the disease.

Small-cell carcinoma (25%)

Small-cell carcinoma is a highly malignant cancer which has usually disseminated widely by the time of diagnosis such that systemic treatment in the form of **chemotherapy** is required. On rare occasions when small-cell carcinoma is diagnosed by surgical resection of a peripheral nodule, adjuvant chemotherapy is given post-operatively. Various combinations of chemotherapeutic agents have been evolved using drugs such as etoposide, carboplatin, cis-platin, cyclophosphamide, adriamycin and vin-cristine. Newer agents being evaluated include gemcitabine and taxol. Combinations of these drugs are usually given as a day treatment in pulses at intervals of about 4 weeks for up to six cycles of treatment. Untreated patients with small-cell carcinoma are usually very symptomatic with a median survival of only 3 months. Combination chemotherapy achieves a symptom-relieving remission of the cancer in about 80% of patients with reduction in tumour size and prolongation of survival to about 11 months. For clinical purposes small-cell cancer is staged as **limited disease** (involving one hemithorax including ipsilateral pleura, hilar or supraclavicular nodes) or **extensive disease** (spread beyond one hemithorax). Patients who have limited stage disease with good general health and who show a good response to chemotherapy have the best prognosis and 5–10% of these patients achieve prolonged survival. After chemo-therapy **consolidation radiotherapy** is usually given to the site of the tumour and mediastinal nodes. Cerebral metastases are common so that prophylactic cranial radio-therapy is sometimes also given. For patients unable to tolerate combination chemotherapy, single-agent oral etoposide may provide useful anti-tumour activity, although it is less effective than combination chemotherapy. Patients receiving chemotherapy require careful moni-toring of their full blood count to avoid prob-lems arising from bone marrow suppression such as anaemia, haemorrhage or infection. Hair loss occurs and patients may choose to wear a wig. Careful attention to anti-emetic medications (e.g. ondansetron, domperidone, metoclopramide) can usually prevent nausea and vomiting.

Non-small-cell cancer (75%)

Surgical resection of the tumour offers the best chance of cure in non-small-cell carci-noma but is only possible if the patient is fit for surgery and if the tumour has not already metastasized. **Staging** (Table 13.2) is the assessment of the extent and spread of the disease and is important in determining the potential resectability of the tumour and the prognosis of the patient. The TNM system is the most widely used and is based upon the size, location and degree of invasion of the tumour (T), the presence of regional lymph node involvement (N) and distant metastases (M). The accuracy of staging depends on the degree of assessment, e.g. staging at thoraco-tomy may show more advanced disease than was apparent on computed tomography (CT) scanning.

When staging a tumour the patient's **symp-toms** should be carefully reviewed for any indication of metastatic disease (e.g. bone pain). Clinical **examination** may show evi-dence of tumour spread to lymph nodes or reveal features of distant metastases. **Bron-choscopy** allows direct visualization of many tumours and may show features of inoperabil-ity (e.g. vocal cord palsy, splaying of the carina by subcarinal lymphadenopathy, or extension of the tumour to within 2 cm of the main carina). Elevated liver function tests or bone **biochemistry** are indications for imaging of the liver by ultrasound or CT scans, and bone by isotope scans. Tumours which appear oper-able should then be assessed by **CT scanning** of the chest, particularly to assess hilar and mediastinal nodes. Enlarged (greater than 1 cm) lymph nodes are suggestive of malignant

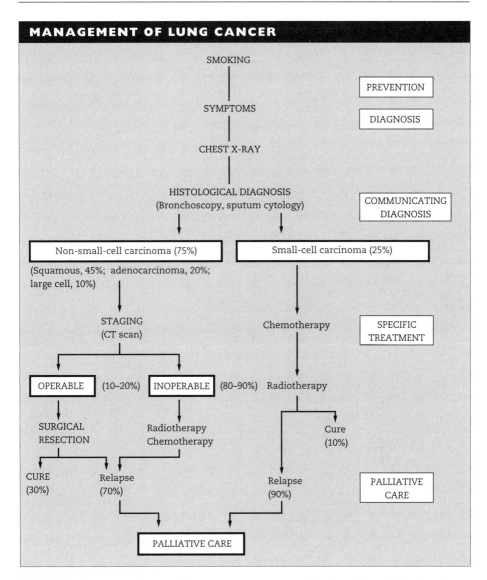

MANAGEMENT OF LUNG CANCER

SMOKING

PREVENTION

SYMPTOMS

DIAGNOSIS

CHEST X-RAY

HISTOLOGICAL DIAGNOSIS
(Bronchoscopy, sputum cytology)

COMMUNICATING
DIAGNOSIS

| Non-small-cell carcinoma (75%) | Small-cell carcinoma (25%) |

(Squamous, 45%; adenocarcinoma, 20%;
large cell, 10%)

STAGING
(CT scan)

Chemotherapy

SPECIFIC
TREATMENT

OPERABLE   (10–20%)   INOPERABLE   (80–90%)   Radiotherapy

SURGICAL   Radiotherapy   Cure
RESECTION   Chemotherapy   (10%)

CURE   Relapse   Relapse   PALLIATIVE
(30%)   (70%)   (90%)   CARE

PALLIATIVE CARE

Fig. 13.7 The 5-year mortality rate of lung cancer is about 90%, emphasizing the fact that the disease is usually disseminated at the time of presentation. Prevention of lung cancer by avoidance of smoking is the most important strategy in the fight against this disease. Choice of treatment depends on cell type and stage of disease. About 25% of lung cancers are small-cell carcinomas and are best treated by chemotherapy followed by radiotherapy. There is usually a good response to chemotherapy but relapse is likely. About 75% are non-small-cell carcinomas and require careful staging and assessment for potential operability. About 10–20% of non-small-cell carcinomas are suitable for surgery but only 30% of patients undergoing resection will be alive in 5 years. A judicious plan of assessment allows careful selection of the best choice of specific anti-cancer treatment with either curative or palliative intent. Symptom relief and palliative care are crucial aspects in the overall management, and the communication of information between doctor and patient at all stages of the disease is of paramount importance.

TNM STAGES

Stage	TNM	Operability	5-year survival (%)
I	$T_{1-2}N_0M_0$		50–60
II	$T_{1-2}N_1M_0$	Operable	30
IIIa	$T_3N_{0-1}M_0$		
	$T_{1-2}N_{2-1}M_0$		20
IIIb	$T_{1-3}N_3M_0$		0
	$T_4N_0M_0$	Inoperable	
IV	Any T, any N, M		0

Tumour (T)
T_1: <3 cm and not involving main bronchus
T_2: >3 cm, or involving main bronchus
T_3: any size, invading chest wall, or within 2 cm of carina
T_4: invading mediastinum, great vessels, trachea

Node (N)
N_0: no regional node metastases
N_1: ipsilateral hilar node metastases
N_2: ipsilateral mediastinal node metastases

Table 13.2 Outline of some TNM stages of non-small-cell carcinoma.

involvement, but if the tumour otherwise appears operable then **mediastinoscopy** is a useful procedure whereby under general anaesthesia, the mediastinum is explored and enlarged nodes biopsied. The decision about the **patient's fitness** to undergo resection of the tumour is based particularly upon the lung function tests and the patient's general fitness. Unfortunately these patients often have substantial cardiovascular disease and smoking-related COPD. No single test predicts feasibility of surgical resection and greater risks may be justified for a tumour which is otherwise curable by resection but a forced expiratory volume in 1 second (FEV_1) <50% of predicted or the presence of hypoxaemia (Po_2 less than 8 kPa (60 mmHg)) would suggest that the patient is not fit for thoracotomy. Unfortunately only about 10–20% of all non-small-cell carcinomas prove suitable for surgery.

Radiotherapy is chiefly undertaken for the relief of symptoms. Superior vena caval obstruction, lobar collapse from bronchial obstruction, haemoptysis or chest wall pain usually respond well to radiotherapy. Radical radiotherapy, using larger doses, is occasionally

used with curative intent for small localized tumours which are not treatable by surgery because of poor patient fitness.

Chemotherapy is being used increasingly for inoperable non-small-cell lung cancer, mainly for palliation of symptoms. A combination of mitomycin C, ifosfamide and cisplatin is usually given in pulses every 3–4 weeks. About 50% of patients with inoperable small-cell carcinoma show a response to chemotherapy with a reduction in tumour size and a median survival of about 10 months.

Palliative care
Palliative care focuses on improving the patient's functioning and psychosocial well-being with relief of symptoms. Even when the disease cannot be cured rapid assessment and diagnosis is important in addressing the patient's symptoms and anxieties. Regular review of patients with lung cancer is essential in providing support for the patient and his or her family and in identifying the nature and origin of symptoms as they arise.

When dealing with a symptom such as pain, specific anti-cancer treatment (e.g. radiotherapy) is often the most effective method of symptom relief. Where there is persistent pain, analgesics need to be given regularly and prophylactically in advance of the return of pain. Mild pain may be treated by a non-opioid analgesic (e.g. a non-steroidal anti-inflammatory drug (NSAID) or paracetamol). More severe pain may be treated by a combination of a weak opioid (e.g. codeine) and a non-opioid (e.g. naproxen) drug. Strong opioids should be used immediately for any severe pain. Often pain control is achieved by use of slow-release morphine tablets (e.g. MST continuous 12 hourly) combined with a NSAID, with additional use of morphine solution for any breakthrough pain. Certain types of pain may benefit from use of co-analgesics such as steroids (e.g. dexamethasone for nerve compression), benzodiazepines (anxiolytic), tricyclic anti-depressants or anti-epileptics (e.g. carbamazepine for neuropathic pain). Whenever opiates are prescribed it is necessary to prescribe a laxative (e.g. co-danthramer) to prevent constipation, and an anti-emetic (e.g. metoclopramide) may be required initially.

Anorexia, weight loss, fatigue and general debility are common in the advanced stages of lung cancer. It is important to check for conditions requiring specific treatment such as anaemia (blood transfusion) or hypercalcaemia (pamidronate). Prednisolone may be useful in boosting appetite, and nutritional supplements may be helpful. Attention needs to be given to the patient's level of social support and help often needs to be given with tasks of daily living. If control of symptoms is not being achieved, help should be sought from a specialist in palliative care.

Other thoracic neoplasms

Alveolar cell carcinoma
This is a rare malignant tumour which arises in the alveoli of the lung and spreads along the alveolar and bronchiolar epithelium. Histologi-

cally it resembles adenocarcinoma. Occasionally this tumour produces large amounts of mucin causing copious sputum production (bronchorrhoea). On chest X-ray it may appear as more diffuse shadowing, resembling pneumonic consolidation, rather than as a discrete mass, and it is sometimes multi-focal in origin. A transbronchial biopsy of alveolar tissue is often necessary for diagnosis. When the tumour is confined to one lobe surgical resection is the treatment of choice.

Carcinoid tumour
This rare tumour is less malignant than bronchial carcinomas in that it rarely metastasizes and is often slow growing, although it may invade locally. It is not related to smoking and often affects younger patients. Most arise in the main bronchi and present with haemoptysis and wheeze. At bronchoscopy the tumour often has a smooth rounded appearance resembling a cherry and it may bleed profusely on biopsy because of its vascularity. Most can be cured by surgical resection. Very rarely a carcinoid tumour of lung metastasizes to the liver where secretion of substances such as 5-hydroxy indoleacetic acid (5-HIAA) produces the carcinoid syndrome of flushing, diarrhoea and wheeze.

Further reading

Carbone DP, Minna JD. Chemotherapy for non-small-cell lung cancer. *BMJ* 1995; **311**: 889–90.
Doll R, Hill AB. The mortality of doctors in relation to their smoking habits. *BMJ* 1954; i: 1451–5.
Hackshaw AK, Law MR, Wald NJ. The accumulated evidence on lung cancer and environmental tobacco smoke. *BMJ* 1997; **315**: 980–8.
Lung and Asthma Information Agency. *Trends in Lung Cancer and Smoking*. Factsheet 93/1.
Osterlind K. Chemotherapy in small-cell lung cancer. *Eur Respir Monogr* 1995; **1**: 306–31.
Sell L, Devlin B, Bourke SJ et al. Communicating the diagnosis of lung cancer. *Respir Med* 1993; **87**: 61–3.

CHAPTER 14

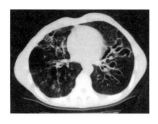

Interstitial Lung Disease

Introduction

Clinical presentation

The terms 'interstitial lung disease' and 'diffuse parenchymal lung disease' are imprecise clinical terms used to refer to a diverse range of diseases which affect the alveoli and septal interstitium of the lung, and which may progress to diffuse lung fibrosis. Patients with these diseases typically present with progressive **dyspnoea**, a dry cough, lung **crackles** and diffuse **infiltrates on chest X-ray**. Lung function tests usually show a restrictive defect (reduced total lung capacity and vital capacity (VC), with normal forced expiratory volume in 1 second/VC (FEV_1/VC) ratio, **impaired gas diffusion** (reduced transfer factor) and **hypoxaemia** with hypocapnia.

Differential diagnosis

Once the clinical features suggest interstitial lung disease a careful search for potential causes is undertaken. Particular attention is paid to any environmental **antigens** (e.g. budgie), **toxins** (e.g. paraquat) or **dusts** (e.g. asbestos) which the patient encounters in his or her **occupational** or **home environment**. **Systemic diseases** (e.g. rheumatoid disease) commonly involve the lung parenchyma and many **drugs** can cause lung fibrosis (e.g. amiodarone, nitrofurantoin, bleomycin) or eosinophilic reactions in the alveoli (e.g. sulphonamides, naproxen). Occasionally there may be difficulties in distinguishing this group of diseases from other causes of diffuse lung infiltrates such as pulmonary oedema, bronchiectasis, and alveolar cell carcinoma. High-resolution computed tomography (CT) gives detailed information about the lung parenchyma and its involvement in a disease process, defining the extent and pattern of the disease.

Investigations

In some cases the clinical assessment allows a diagnosis to be made with reasonable certainty but it is often useful to obtain a biopsy of the lung parenchyma for histology. Small samples can be obtained by **transbronchial biopsy** of the lung parenchyma through a flexible bronchoscope (Fig. 14.1). Larger samples can be obtained by **surgical biopsy** under general anaesthesia either by **thoracotomy** or by **video-assisted thoracoscopy**. In many cases the histological features are characteristic of a particular disease (e.g. granulomas in sarcoidosis or extrinsic allergic alveolitis; tumour cells in lymphangitis carcinomatosa), but in advanced disease the histology may show non-specific lung fibrosis without clues to its aetiology. **Bronchoalveolar lavage** may be performed through the bronchoscope at the same time as transbronchial biopsy. Aliquots of saline are instilled via the bronchoscope which is held in a wedged position in a

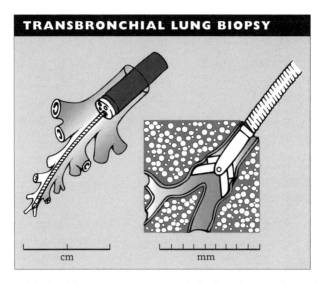

TRANSBRONCHIAL LUNG BIOPSY

cm   mm

Fig. 14.1 Transbronchial lung biopsy: A small specimen of lung parenchyma can be obtained by passing a biopsy forceps through a flexible bronchoscope, usually under radiological guidance, into the lung periphery. A sample of lung tissue is obtained by biopsying between two limbs in a branching small bronchus. There is a small risk of causing haemorrhage or pneumothorax, so the patient's condition and lung function should be adequate to tolerate these complications.

subsegmental bronchus, and fluid is then aspirated for cell analysis. A lymphocytic alveolitis is characteristic of sarcoidosis, for example. Many of these diseases are characterized in their early stages by an inflammatory alveolitis, which is responsive to corticosteroids, whereas in the later stages there may be irreversible lung fibrosis.

Careful clinical investigation of patients presenting with features of interstitial lung disease aims to move from this imprecise clinical label to a diagnosis of a specific disease process (Fig. 14.2).

Cryptogenic fibrosing alveolitis

Cryptogenic fibrosing alveolitis (idiopathic pulmonary fibrosis) is a serious disease which kills about 1000 people each year in the UK. It is more common in men (**male/female ratio 2 : 1**) and in the elderly (**mean age 67 years**). It presents with the typical features of an interstitial lung disease as progressive **dyspnoea**, dry cough, **crackles**, restrictive defect in lung function and reticulonodular **infiltrates on chest X-ray** (Fig. 14.3). About 50% have **clubbing**. The aetiology is unknown but the disease probably represents the inflammatory and immune response of the lung to tissue damage. A possible association with previous exposure to environmental dusts (e.g. metal or wood dust) has been found in some epidemiological studies, and about 30% of patients have autoantibodies (e.g. rheumatoid factor, anti-nuclear factor) in their serum. The diagnosis is often made on the basis of the clinical features but lung biopsy helps to confirm the diagnosis, to exclude other causes, and to give information about the stage of the disease. The typical **histological features** are cellular thickening of the alveolar walls with fibrosis and an inflammatory cell infiltrate in the alveoli. These features have been classified in various ways but from a clinical point of view the degrees of cellularity and fibrosis are the most important.

INTERSTITIAL LUNG DISEASE

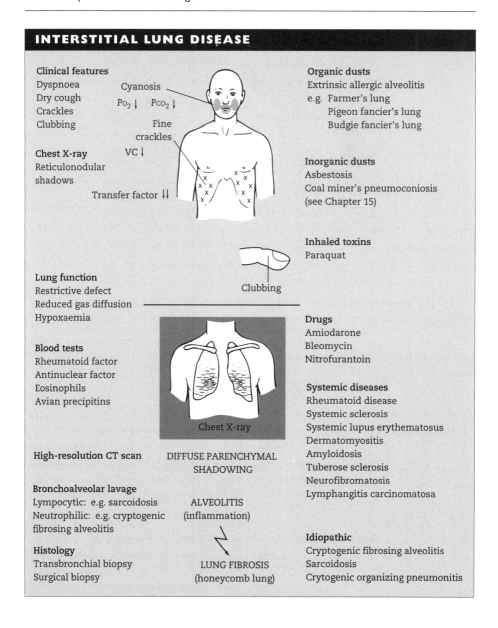

Clinical features
Dyspnoea   Cyanosis
Dry cough $Po_2 \downarrow$ $Pco_2 \downarrow$
Crackles
Clubbing   Fine
                 crackles

Chest X-ray   VC $\downarrow$
Reticulonodular
shadows
         Transfer factor $\downarrow\downarrow$

Lung function
Restrictive defect
Reduced gas diffusion
Hypoxaemia

Blood tests
Rheumatoid factor
Antinuclear factor
Eosinophils
Avian precipitins

High-resolution CT scan   DIFFUSE PARENCHYMAL
                               SHADOWING

Bronchoalveolar lavage
Lympocytic: e.g. sarcoidosis   ALVEOLITIS
Neutrophilic: e.g. cryptogenic   (inflammation)
fibrosing alveolitis

Histology
Transbronchial biopsy   LUNG FIBROSIS
Surgical biopsy   (honeycomb lung)

Clubbing

Chest X-ray

Organic dusts
Extrinsic allergic alveolitis
e.g. Farmer's lung
     Pigeon fancier's lung
     Budgie fancier's lung

Inorganic dusts
Asbestosis
Coal miner's pneumoconiosis
(see Chapter 15)

Inhaled toxins
Paraquat

Drugs
Amiodarone
Bleomycin
Nitrofurantoin

Systemic diseases
Rheumatoid disease
Systemic sclerosis
Systemic lupus erythematosus
Dermatomyositis
Amyloidosis
Tuberose sclerosis
Neurofibromatosis
Lymphangitis carcinomatosa

Idiopathic
Cryptogenic fibrosing alveolitis
Sarcoidosis
Crytogenic organizing pneumonitis

Fig. 14.2 Summary of the clinical investigations and differential diagnosis of interstitial lung disease.

Patients with a **cellular pattern** (i.e. predominantly inflammatory cellular infiltrate with little fibrosis) are probably in an earlier stage of the disease and show a better response to steroids than patients with a **fibrotic pattern**. A 'ground glass' appearance on **high-resolution CT scan** corresponds to the cellular pattern on histology whereas a 'reticular' pattern indicates fibrosis.

The clinical course of the disease is very variable with some patients following an indolent course over many years whereas others

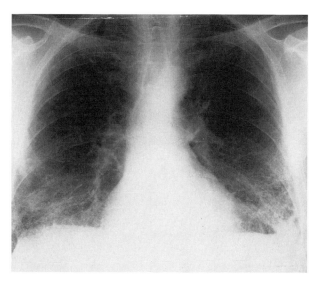

Fig. 14.3 This 70-year-old man presented with a 6-month history of progressive breathlessness, crackles and clubbing with reduced lung volumes and impaired gas diffusion. The chest X-ray shows small lung volumes with reticular shadowing particularly affecting the lung peripheries and bases suggesting cryptogenic fibrosing alveolitis. He failed to respond to prednisolone and died 1 year later of respiratory failure.

show a rapid progression. Overall about **50% of patients die within 3 years** of diagnosis. High-dose **corticosteroids** (e.g. prednisolone 60 mg/day) are the main treatment but only about 20–30% of patients show a good response. Usually any response will be apparent within 1–2 months at which stage the benefits and side-effects of prolonged steroid treatment must be carefully considered. **Cyclophosphamide** or **azathioprine** are second-line treatments which may be tried where there is no response to steroids. For younger patients **lung transplantation** may be an option (see Chapter 20).

Connective tissue diseases

In about 35% of cases the typical features of cryptogenic fibrosing alveolitis occur in association with a connective tissue disease. These diseases have a number of other lung complications.

Rheumatoid disease (Fig. 14.4)

Involvement of the **cricoarytenoid joint** causes hoarseness and sometimes stridor. **Obliterative bronchiolitis** results in progressive peripheral airways obstruction. **Pleural effusions** are common and analysis of the pleural fluid characteristically shows a high protein level (exudate) with a low glucose concentration and a high titre of rheumatoid factor. **Rheumatoid nodules** may develop in the lung parenchyma and show the same histological features as the rheumatoid subcutaneous nodules. When rheumatoid disease occurs in association with coalworker's pneumoconiosis, large cavitating pulmonary nodules may develop **(Caplan's syndrome)**. **Drugs** (e.g. gold, penicillamine) used to treat rheumatoid disease may cause lung fibrosis. **Fibrosing alveolitis** complicating rheumatoid disease is managed in the same way as 'lone' cryptogenic fibrosing alveolitis.

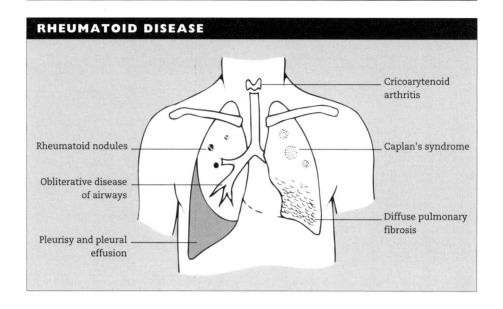

RHEUMATOID DISEASE

Cricoarytenoid arthritis

Rheumatoid nodules

Caplan's syndrome

Obliterative disease of airways

Diffuse pulmonary fibrosis

Pleurisy and pleural effusion

Fig. 14.4 Summary of pulmonary complications of rheumatoid disease.

Systemic sclerosis (scleroderma)

Diffuse **fibrosing alveolitis** is the most common complication. **Pulmonary vasculitis** with pulmonary hypertension and cor pulmonale may occur. **Chest wall restriction** by contraction of the skin is rare. **Aspiration pneumonia** may occur due to oesophageal dysmotility in the CREST variant of the disease: calcinosis, Raynaud's phenomenon, oesophageal dysfunction, sclerodactyly and telangiectasia.

Systemic lupus erythematosus

Pleural effusions are common and may cause **pleural thickening**. The phenomenon of **'shrinking lungs'**, in which the chest X-ray shows high hemidiaphragms with small lungs, is probably due to myopathy of the diaphragm. **Fibrosing alveolitis** may occur. Immunosuppressive treatments predispose to **opportunistic infections** (e.g. *Pneumocystis carinii*).

Cryptogenic organizing pneumonitis

Cryptogenic organizing pneumonitis (COP) (or bronchiolitis obliterans organizing pneumonia (BOOP)) is an uncommon condition characterized by the occurrence of **intra-alveolar buds of organizing fibrosis** with obliteration of bronchioles on lung biopsy. It seems to be a pattern of response in the lungs to a variety of insults. It particularly occurs in association with some **drugs** (e.g. amiodarone, sulphasalazine, gold), **connective tissue diseases** (e.g. rheumatoid disease) or ulcerative colitis, and **often no cause is identifiable**. Clinically patients often have cough, malaise, fever, dyspnoea with chest X-ray infiltrates and elevated erythrocyte sedimentation rate (ESR). Often the patient is thought to have infective pneumonia but the differential diagnosis is widened when no pathogen is identified and the patient fails to respond to antibiotics. A range of **chest X-ray** abnormalities occur including **fleeting shadows**, localized **alveolar infiltrates** and diffuse **reticular shadowing**. Since the same histological pattern is found as a result of a variety of insults to the lung 'BOOP/COP' is probably not a single entity but one pattern of response of the lungs to injury. Characteristically there is a **dramatic response to corticosteroids** although relapse may occur as the dose is reduced.

Extrinsic allergic alveolitis

Extrinsic allergic alveolitis (hypersensitivity pneumonitis) is an **immunologically mediated lung disease** in which a hypersensitivity response occurs in a **sensitized individual** to an **inhaled antigen**. Typical examples of this disease are **farmer's lung** and **bird fancier's lung**. When hay is harvested and stored in damp conditions it becomes mouldy, generating heat which encourages growth of fungi such as *Thermoactinomyces vulgaris* or *Micropolyspora faeni*. When the hay is subsequently used for foddering cattle, fungal spores may be inhaled. Avian antigens are inhaled by people who participate in the sport of pigeon racing or who keep pet birds such as budgies. The inhalation of these antigens provokes a complex immune response in susceptible subjects involving antibody reactions, immune-complex formation, complement activation and cellular responses, resulting in alveolitis. Strangely these diseases are less common in smokers.

In the **acute form** of the disease the patient typically experiences recurrent episodes of dyspnoea, dry cough, pyrexia, myalgia, and a flu-like sensation, occurring about 4–8 hours after antigen exposure. During such an episode lung function tests may show a reduction in lung volumes and gas diffusion, and chest X-ray may show diffuse shadowing. The acute illness is often misdiagnosed as a pneumonia. The **chronic form** is characterized by the insidious development of dyspnoea and lung fibrosis. Lung biopsies show features of fibrosis, alveolitis and granuloma formation. Bronchoalveolar lavage typically shows evidence of a lymphocytic alveolitis with a predominance of T-suppressor lymphocytes. Precipitating anti-

bodies to avian or fungal antigens can be detected in serum but are also found in many asymptomatic subjects so that they are not diagnostic.

Complete **cessation of exposure to the provoking antigen** is the main treatment. However, pigeon fanciers, for example, are very committed to their sport and will often wish to continue keeping pigeons. They can reduce antigen contact by wearing a mask and a loft-coat and hat (so as to avoid carrying antigen on their clothing or hair). **Steroids** (e.g. prednisolone 40 mg/day) hasten the resolution of the alveolitis and are often used during severe acute episodes. The immune response in extrinsic allergic alveolitis is complex and a variety of modulating factors influence the interaction of antigenic stimulus and host response so that the longitudinal course of the disease is variable with some patients developing lung fibrosis and others showing spontaneous improvement despite continued antigen exposure.

Sarcoidosis

Sarcoidosis is a mysterious **multi-system disease** characterized by the occurrence in affected organs of **non-caseating granulomatous lesions** which may progress to cause fibrosis. The aetiology is unknown but the accumulation of T4-helper lymphocytes at disease sites is suggestive of an immunological reaction to an unidentified poorly degradable antigen. The frequent involvement of the lungs raises the possibility that such a putative antigen enters the body via the lungs. The compartmentalization of T4 lymphocytes in affected tissues is associated with a corresponding depletion of T4 cells in other tissues and depression of some delayed-type hypersensitivity responses such that patients with sarcoidosis often demonstrate negative reactions to tuberculin (i.e. negative Heaf or Mantoux tests despite previous bacillus Calmette–Guérin (BCG) vaccination). Serum immunoglobulin levels are usually elevated and

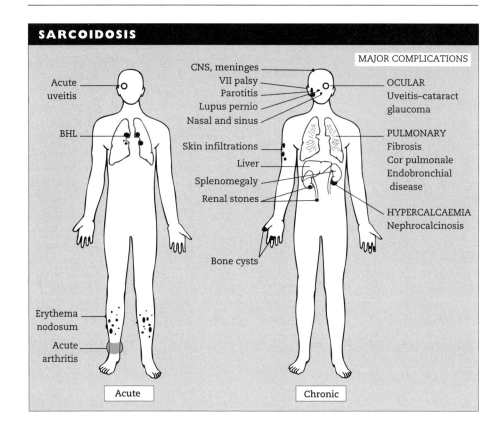

Fig. 14.5 Principal clinical features of sarcoidosis. BHL, bilateral hilar lymphadenopathy.

immune complexes are often present in acute sarcoidosis.

The clinical features of sarcoidosis are very varied but it is useful to consider two broad categories of disease: an acute form which is usually transient and often resolves spontaneously and a chronic form which is persistent and may cause fibrosis (Fig. 14.5).

Acute sarcoidosis

The acute form typically develops abruptly in young adults with **erythema nodosum** and **bilateral hilar lymphadenopathy** sometimes with **uveitis**, **arthritis** and **parotitis**.

Erythema nodosum

This appears as **round, red, raised nodules** typically over the shins. It is a manifestation of hypersensitivity and is also found in other diseases such as streptococcal infection, tuberculosis, ulcerative colitis and Crohn's disease, and with drugs (e.g. sulphonamides, contraceptive pill), but in many cases no cause is identified.

Bilateral hilar lymphadenopathy

Bilateral hilar lymphadenopathy (BHL) is not associated with any signs on examination of the chest or with any loss of lung function and is often found incidentally on a **chest X-ray**, but often the X-ray was taken in a patient with other features suggestive of sarcoidosis (Fig. 14.6). Although sarcoidosis is the most important cause of BHL other causes include lym-

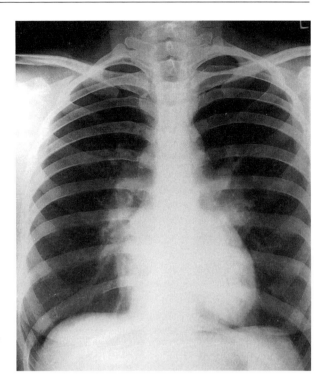

Fig. 14.6 This 25-year-old woman presented with uveitis, arthralgia and erythema nodosum of her shins. The chest X-ray shows bilateral hilar lymphadenopathy. She was otherwise well and lung function tests were normal. A diagnosis of probable acute sarcoidosis was made. The disease resolved spontaneously without the need for any medical intervention.

phoma, metastatic carcinoma, tuberculosis, fungal infections such as coccidioidomycosis and histoplasmosis in endemic areas (e.g. North America); and, in the past berylliosis (e.g. beryllium used in fluorescent lighting).

Chronic sarcoidosis

The chronic form of sarcoidosis pursues a more indolent course, often in an older age group, with involvement of many tissues of the body.

Chronic pulmonary sarcoidosis

This involves the lung parenchyma with **reticular shadowing** often distributed in a perihilar fashion on chest X-ray (Fig. 14.7). There are often remarkably few signs on examination of the chest, and lung function may be well maintained but the disease may progress in some patients causing **progressive fibrosis** and loss of lung function with impairment of gas diffusion, reduction in lung volumes and sometimes airways obstruction with air trapping and bulla formation.

Chronic extrapulmonary sarcoidosis

Sarcoidosis may affect virtually any organ in the body. **Ocular sarcoidosis** often presents as pain and redness of the eye due to anterior uveitis. Chorioretinitis, keratoconjunctivitis sicca and lacrimal gland enlargement may complicate chronic sarcoidosis. **Parotid gland enlargement** may be painful and sometimes causes facial nerve palsy. **Central nervous system** involvement may cause cranial nerve palsies, chronic meningitis, obstructive hydrocephalus and a variety of neurological syndromes. **Posterior pituitary** involvement may rarely cause diabetes insipidus. **Cutaneous sarcoidosis** may cause maculopapular eruptions, plaques, nodules and lupus pernio (a violaceous chronic skin lesion particularly affecting the nose and cheeks). **Bone** cysts are sometimes found and are often asymptomatic.

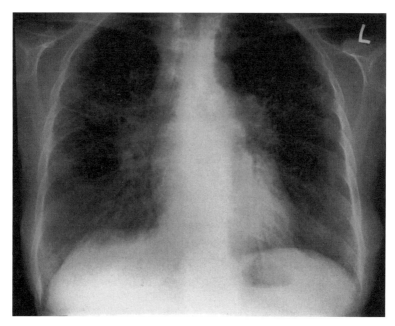

Fig. 14.7 This 60-year-old woman presented with cough and progressive breathlessness. There were no crackles on auscultation of her chest but transfer factor for carbon monoxide and transfer coefficient were reduced to 60% of the predicted values. The chest X-ray shows extensive perihilar reticular shadowing. Transbronchial lung biopsy showed non-caseating granulomas and lung fibrosis. Tests for tuberculosis were negative. She was treated with prednisolone with some improvement in lung function.

Cardiac sarcoid may cause conduction system damage and arrhythmias. **Hypercalcaemia** may result from increased bone resorption, and nephrocalcinosis, hypercalcuria and renal calculi may occur. Sarcoid granulomas and fibrosis may also be found in the liver, spleen, lymph nodes and muscle, for example.

Diagnosis

The diagnosis of sarcoidosis can often be made on **clinical** grounds particularly when a young adult presents with classic features such as erythema nodosum and BHL. In less typical cases it is helpful to obtain **biopsy of an affected organ**. **Transbronchial biopsy** is particularly useful and may be combined with **bronchoalveolar lavage**, which typically demonstrates evidence of a T4-helper lymphocyte alveolitis. **Mediastinoscopy** and biopsy of hilar lymph nodes is sometimes indicated to exclude other diagnoses such as lymphoma.

The Kveim test is useful where there is doubt about the diagnosis and where no other tissue is accessible to biopsy. It consists of the intradermal injection of an extract of human sarcoid spleen with biopsy of the injection site 6 weeks later. A positive result is indicated by the presence of sarcoid granuloma. There is a potential hazard of transmission of unknown factors (e.g. slow viruses, prions) in the injection of splenic tissue from person to person, although no such adverse reaction has been reported. The histological appearances must be considered in the clinical context since they are not in themselves diagnostic, and other granulomatous disease (e.g. tuberculosis) must be excluded. Serum angiotensin-converting enzyme (ACE) levels are elevated in about two-thirds of patients with active sarcoidosis but this test lacks sensitivity and specificity and is therefore of limited value in diagnosis, or in monitoring the course of the disease.

Treatment

In most patients sarcoidosis is a **self-limiting disease** which **resolves spontaneously** without treatment. However, a minority of patients with chronic sarcoidosis develop progressive fibrosis. Since the cause of sarcoidosis is unknown no specific treatment is available but **corticosteroids** suppress inflammation in the affected organs frequently improving local and systemic symptoms. Their effect on the long-term natural history of sarcoidosis is less clear. They are usually used in patients with progressive disease and studies suggest some benefit from steroid therapy at the cost of side-effects (e.g. osteoporosis, Cushing's syndrome). A short course of prednisolone is sometimes used for particularly troublesome acute symptoms such as parotitis, arthritis or erythema nodosum if non-steroidal anti-inflammatory drugs are not sufficient. Uveitis may be treated by topical steroids, and skin manifestations may be amenable to steroid creams or steroid injections. Inhaled steroids have been tried for pulmonary disease but evidence of efficacy is lacking. In chronic sarcoidosis deciding who to treat and when to treat requires **careful judgement to balance the benefit and risks of chronic steroid therapy**.

Further reading

Bourke SJ, Boyd G. Pigeon fancier's lung. *BMJ* 1997; **315**: 70–1.

Evans CC. Rheumatic and connective tissue diseases. In: Brewis RAL, Corrin B, Geddes DM, Gibson GJ, eds. *Respiratory Medicine*. London: WB Saunders Co, 1995: 1673–85.

Geddes DM. BOOP and COP. *Thorax* 1991; **46**: 545–7.

Johnston IDA, Prescott RJ, Chalmers JC, Rudd RM. British Thoracic Society Study of cryptogenic fibrosing alveolitis: Current presentation and initial management. *Thorax* 1997; **52**: 38–44.

O'Connor CM, Fitzgerald MX. Speculations on sarcoidosis. *Respir Med* 1992; **86**: 277–82.

CHAPTER 15

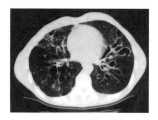

Occupational Lung Disease

Introduction

The importance of the work environment as a cause of lung disease has been recognized since ancient times. Hippocrates (460–377 BC) taught his pupils to observe the environment of their patients. Ramazzini urged physicians to ask patients what work they did and to visit the workplace. In 1713 he published a treatise on work-related diseases (*De Morbis Artificium*) which included descriptions of baker's asthma and what is now known as extrinsic allergic alveolitis. Occupational lung diseases result from the inhalation of dusts, gases, fumes or vapours encountered in the workplace, and the hazards of the work environment are constantly changing as old industries are replaced by new ones. The effects of inhaled substances depend on many factors including particle size, physical characteristics (e.g. solubility), toxicity, the intensity and duration of exposures, and the person's susceptibility. Particles $>10\,\mu m$ in diameter are usually filtered out of the inhaled airstream in the nose; particles of $1–10\,\mu m$ are mainly deposited in the bronchi; and particles $<1\,\mu m$ penetrate to the alveoli. Inhaled substances may exert their effects in various ways, and in many circumstances the precise mechanisms involved are incompletely understood. Some substances exert a non-specific **irritant** effect (e.g. generally dusty environment) or are **toxic** to the airways (e.g. chlorine, ammonia) with all workers exposed being similarly affected. Other substances induce **hypersensitivity** or allergic reactions in susceptible individuals giving rise to asthma or extrinsic allergic alveolitis (see Chapter 14), for example. Some inhaled dusts **promote fibrosis** in the lung parenchyma (e.g. silica, asbestos, coal dust) and some are **carcinogenic** (e.g. cigarette smoke, asbestos). Occasionally **infective organisms** are inhaled (e.g. *Mycobacterium tuberculosis* in health-care workers, *Chlamydia psittaci* in bird handlers).

Occupational asthma

Asthma is now the most common type of occupational lung disease. Occupational asthma may be defined as **variable airways obstruction caused by a sensitizing agent inhaled at work**. This definition excludes the triggering of episodes of wheezing in patients with pre-existing asthma by irritant mechanisms such as cold air or exercise at work. The list of causes of occupational asthma is long and new agents are being continuously added. Some of the most common causes are shown in Table 15.1. Occupational asthma is rare amongst library, professional and clerical workers but is common amongst spray painters (isocyanates), bakers (flour), hairdressers (persulphates) and workers in the

CAUSES OF OCCUPATIONAL ASTHMA

Agent	Occupational exposure
Isocyanates	Spray paints, varnishes, adhesives, polyurethane foam manufacture
Flour	Bakers
Colophony	Electronic soldering flux
Epoxy resins	Hardening agents, adhesives
Animals (rats, mice)	Laboratory workers
Wood dusts	Sawmill workers, joiners
Azodicarbonamide	Polyvinyl plastics manufacture
Persulphate salts	Hairdressers
Drugs (penicillin, cephalosporins)	Pharmaceutical industry
Grain dust (mites, moulds)	Farmers, millers, bakers

Table 15.1 Common causes of occupational asthma.

plastics and chemical industries (epoxy resins, azodicarbonamide), for example.

Diagnosis

To establish a diagnosis of occupational asthma it is first necessary to **confirm the presence of asthma** and secondly to show a **causal relationship between the asthma and the work environment**. Although the suspicion of occupational asthma is often based upon the **patient's history** the diagnosis should be confirmed by **objective tests** wherever possible because of the importance of the diagnosis in terms of managing the patient, identifying the causative agent, reducing the risk to other workers and addressing the medicolegal and compensation aspects of the diagnosis.

Characteristically there is an initial asymptomatic period of exposure to the agent before symptoms develop. This **latent interval** varies from a few weeks to several years. Once the worker has developed sensitization to the agent further exposure may provoke an **early asthmatic response** (reaching a peak within 30 minutes), a **late asthmatic response** (occurring 4–12 hours later) or a **dual response**. If an early response occurs, the relationship of symptoms to the work environment is usually apparent. Late responses typi-

cally develop the evening after exposure, disturbing sleep and causing cough and wheeze the following morning. Initially symptoms **improve away from work** on holidays or at weekends and **deteriorate on return to work**. Once asthma becomes established symptoms may persist even when away from the work environment and are also triggered by other factors such as exercise or cold air. Sometimes the sensitizing agent also causes rhinitis and dermatitis. Occupational asthma may develop in workers with pre-existing asthma and this may lead to a delay in diagnosis if the relationship of symptoms to the work environment is not recognized. The patient may be exposed to a known inducer of asthma (e.g. paint sprayers using isocyanates) but doctors need to be constantly alert to new causes of occupational asthma.

Serial measurement of **peak expiratory flow** or **spirometry** over several days at work and away from work will usually show evidence of variable airways obstruction (the hallmark of asthma) and may demonstrate a relationship between symptoms, airways obstruction and the work environment. Lung function tests may be normal when the patient is seen away from the work environment. Assessment and management of occupational asthma is notoriously difficult as some workers may be reluctant to admit to symptoms in case this jeopardises their employment. Conversely others may exaggerate symptoms in an attempt to gain compensation. Patients with suspected occupational asthma should therefore be referred for specialist assessment. One of the best ways of showing a relationship between asthma and the work environment is to perform a carefully supervised **workplace challenge study**. In this the patient is removed from the work environment for about 2 weeks and then returned to work under supervision. Serial measurements of spirometry or peak expiratory flow are performed on control days away from work and then over about 3 days on return to the patient's normal work environment. Serial measurements of **airway responsiveness** to methacholine or histamine (see Chapter 11) typically show sequential improvement away from work and rapid deterioration on return to work. Figure 15.1 shows a typical late asth-

matic reaction occurring during a workplace challenge study in a worker in a biocide manufacturing plant. The agent inducing the patient's asthma can often be identified with reasonable confidence by a **visit to the workplace** and an assessment of the materials used. However, workers may be exposed to many agents and it may be difficult to know which agent is causing asthma. **Laboratory challenge studies** involve the patient inhaling the specific suspect agent under double-blind, carefully controlled circumstances with serial measurements of spirometry and airway responsiveness. These studies are particularly useful in identifying previously unrecognized causes of occupational asthma but they should only be undertaken in specialist units as they are potentially hazardous. In some cases of occupational asthma it is possible to demonstrate a positive skin prick test or circulating antibodies to the agent but such immunological reactions are often present in asymptomatic workers also.

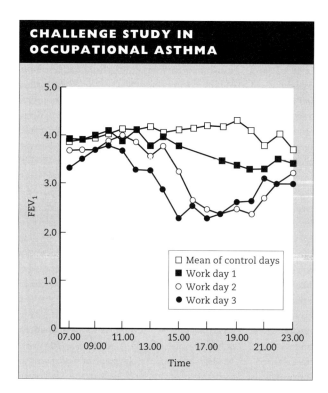

Fig. 15.1 Workplace challenge study showing the mean forced expiratory volume in 1 second (FEV_1) on control days away from the workplace and progressive falls in FEV_1 over 3 days at work indicating late asthmatic reactions of increasing severity occurring in relation to exposure to a biocide in the workplace.

Management

Treatment of occupational asthma involves management of both the **affected individual** and the **affected industry**. Early cessation of exposure to the inducing agent may result in complete resolution of the patient's asthma. The key factor in the patient's treatment is therefore not the institution of bronchodilator and steroid treatments as in conventional asthma but the **avoidance of exposure** to the inducing agent. This may be achieved in a number of ways but often involves moving the patient to a different job within the factory. Where there has been a delay in recognizing the nature of the patient's asthma and in ceasing exposure chronic asthma may develop which persists even after cessation of contact with the inducing agent, and long-term inhaled steroid and bronchodilators drugs are then required.

Substitution of an alternative, non-asthmagenic substance in the industrial process is the ideal solution as this also removes the risk to other workers. Where this is not possible, **enclosure** of the process in a confined booth with **exhaust ventilation** may be possible. **Segregation** of the hazardous process may be useful in limiting the exposure to a small group of workers who are then provided with appropriate personal **protective devices** such as respirator masks. **Surveillance** of other workers should be undertaken where a work environment has been shown to cause asthma. This typically involves a pre-employment medical examination combined with periodic assessment of asthma symptoms, spirometry, and ideally serial measurements of airway responsiveness. Institution of these measures in the workplace requires the cooperation of the factory safety officer, management, occupational health department and industrial hygienist. Hazards within the workplace fall within the remit of governmental agencies such as the Employment Medical Advisory Service (EMAS) of the Health and Safety Executive in the UK. Workers suffering disability as a result of their employment are entitled to **compensation** from the Department of Social Security in the UK, and may also wish to pursue legal action against their employer.

Byssinosis

Byssinosis is a disease of the airway caused by the inhalation of **cotton** or **flax** dust. Symptoms typically arise after several years of working in the industry and show a characteristic pattern different from that seen in occupational asthma. Characteristically workers complain of **chest tightness**, **cough** and **dyspnoea** on Mondays (or the first shift of the week) and, peculiarly, symptoms **improve throughout the working week**. There is sometimes a fall in forced expiratory volume in 1 second (FEV_1) during the working day but there is often a poor correlation between symptoms and FEV_1. Chronic productive cough and irreversible airways obstruction sometimes develop. It is difficult to understand what mechanisms give rise to the pattern of symptoms being worse at the start of the week and improving thereafter. It has been suggested that cotton particles may cause direct release of histamine and that symptoms resolve as histamine stores are depleted. However, the pathogenesis of byssinosis is uncertain, and alternative theories suggest that symptoms may be related to contamination of cotton by Gram-negative bacteria and endotoxins, or that immunological mechanisms may be important.

Pneumoconiosis

Pneumoconiosis is a general term used to describe lung fibrosis resulting from inhalation of dusts such as coal, silica or asbestos.

Coalworker's pneumoconiosis

The development of pneumoconiosis is directly related to the total exposure to coal dust. Dust exposure varies in different parts of the coal mine and is heaviest at the coal face. Improvements in ventilation and working conditions have considerably reduced the level of dust in modern coalmines. In many countries there has been a decline in the coal industry with increased use of alternative sources of energy. In the UK the number of coalminers has fallen from about 750 000 to 20 000 over the last 50 years. Coal dust inhaled into the alveoli is taken up by macrophages which are then cleared via the lymphatic drainage system or via the mucociliary escalator of the bronchial tree. If there is heavy prolonged exposure to dust the clearance mechanisms are overwhelmed and dust macules arise particularly in the region of the respiratory bronchioles. Release of dust from dying macrophages induces fibroblast proliferation and fibrosis. There is an important distinction to be made between the two major categories of coalworker's pneumoconiosis.

• *Simple coalworker's pneumoconiosis* consists of the accumulation, within the lung tissue, of small (<5 mm) aggregations of coal particles which are uniformly dispersed and evident on chest X-ray as a delicate micronodular mottling. **Simple pneumoconiosis is not associated with any significant symptoms, signs, impairment of lung function or alteration to prognosis, e.g. life expectancy.** The size and extent of the nodules can be categorized for research and classification purposes by comparing the patient's X-ray with standard films published by the International Labour Office. The benign nature of simple pneumoconiosis is sometimes not appreciated and there is often a tendency to attribute any respiratory symptoms to the pneumoconiosis, whereas alternative explanations such as chronic obstructive pulmonary disease (COPD), asthma or heart disease are more likely to account for the patient's symptoms.

• *Complicated coalworker's pneumoconiosis* (progressive massive fibrosis) is characterized by the occurrence of large black fibrotic masses in the lung parenchyma, consisting of coal dust and bundles of collagen. These are typically situated in the upper zones and appear as rather **bizarre opacities on chest X-ray** against the background of simple pneumoconiosis (Fig. 15.2). **Cavitation** of these lesions may occur and may result in the expectoration of black sputum (melanoptysis). Complicated pneumoconiosis often results in dyspnoea, a **restrictive ventilatory defect** (reduced lung volumes) and **impaired gas diffusion** (reduced transfer factor for carbon monoxide), and **reduced life expectancy**.

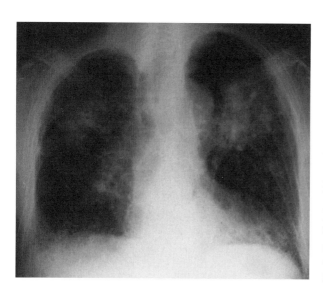

Fig. 15.2 This 78-year-old man, who had been a faceworker in a coalmine for 40 years, presented with progressive breathlessness. Chest X-ray shows irregular opacities of progressive massive fibrosis in both upper lobes with extensive background nodular shadowing of coalworker's pneumoconiosis.

Caplan's syndrome (rheumatoid pneumoconiosis)

Coalworkers with **rheumatoid arthritis** may develop **multiple nodules** of about 0.5–2 cm in diameter in the lungs. These lung nodules are often accompanied by the occurrence of subcutaneous rheumatoid nodules.

Coalworker's bronchitis and emphysema

Coalminers have a high prevalence of **bronchitis**, **airways obstruction** and **emphysema**. This is generally due to **cigarette smoking** but studies suggest that coal dust also contributes to the development of bronchitis and emphysema, and in 1993 the Department of Social Security in the UK decided that coalminers who had spent 20 years or more in underground work and who had reduced FEV_1 were entitled to compensation.

Silicosis

This is a form of pneumoconiosis resulting from the inhalation of free silica (silicon dioxide). It is now uncommon in developed countries because of widespread recognition and control of the hazards of respirable silica dust, but it still occurs in developing countries. There is a risk of silicosis in workers involved in: **quarrying**, grinding and dressing of sandstone, granite and slate; developing **tunnels** and sinking shafts (e.g. coalmines); **boiler scaling**; **sandblasting** of castings in iron and steel foundries; and the **pottery** industry where silica may be used in the lining of kilns and the dry-grinding of ceramic products.

Simple nodular silicosis, like simple coalworker's pneumoconiosis, causes no symptoms and is an X-ray phenomenon. Complicated silicosis, however, results in **progressive fibrosis**, loss of lung function and dyspnoea. The silicotic nodule consists of concentric layers of collagen surrounding a central area of dust including quartz crystals and dying macrophages. There is a significantly increased risk of **tuberculosis** in patients with silicosis

as silica interferes with the ability of macrophages to kill tubercle bacilli. Patients with silicosis are also at increased risk of developing **lung cancer**.

A chest X-ray typically shows **nodular opacities** particularly affecting the **upper lobes**. The nodules are usually denser and larger than those seen in simple coalworker's pneumoconiosis. **Eggshell calcification** of **hilar lymph nodes** is a particularly characteristic feature (Fig. 15.3). **Pleural thickening** may also occur.

Siderosis

Dust containing **iron** and its oxides is encountered at various stages in the iron and steel industry and in welding. It gives rise to a simple pneumoconiosis (siderosis) which produces a striking mottled appearance on the chest X-ray because of the high radiodensity of iron, but which is not accompanied by symptoms, signs or any physiological defect. Other metals such as antimony and tin may produce a similar picture.

Asbestos-related lung disease

Asbestos is a collective term for a number of naturally occurring fibrous mineral silicates which are widely used because of their fire-resistant and insulation properties. Asbestos fibres are of two main types which have different physical and chemical properties: *serpentine asbestos fibres* (**chrysotile—white asbestos**) are wispy, flexible and relatively long such that they are less easily inhaled to the periphery of the lung. *Amphibole asbestos fibres* (e.g. **crocidolite — blue asbestos, amosite — brown asbestos, tremolite**) are straighter, stiffer and more brittle, and penetrate more deeply into the lung. They are also more resistant to breakdown within the lung.

Workers may be exposed to asbestos in many different settings so that it is important to take a detailed history of all the patient's

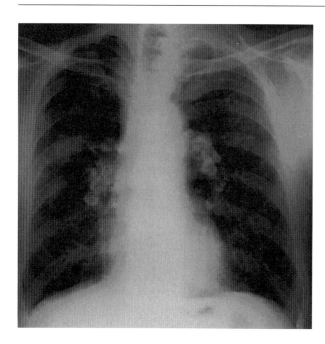

Fig. 15.3 This 65-year-old man had had extensive exposure to silica when working in a stone quarry. Chest X-ray shows eggshell calcification (a rim of calcification around the outer margin) of the hilar lymph nodes with upper lobe fibrosis. Tests for tuberculosis were negative.

occupations over the years and of the tasks undertaken. **Pipe laggers** and industrial **plumbers** often have had heavy exposure to asbestos since it is widely used for **thermal insulation** in **ships**, **power stations** and factories. Many workers in the **shipbuilding** industry were heavily exposed to asbestos when they worked alongside pipe laggers in confined spaces such as the engine rooms of ships. Sometimes housewives washing their husband's work overalls inhaled significant amounts of asbestos. Workers in the **insulation industry** and those producing **asbestos products** may have been heavily exposed. Chrysotile asbestos is used in **brake-pad linings**, in **cement products**, in **pipes, tiles** and **roofing** materials. In many circumstances the asbestos is safely bound within composite materials but respirable dust may be produced by the **cutting of asbestos sheets**, or in demolition work involving the removal, or **stripping-off**, of asbestos insulation from pipes or boilers.

Strict precautions were eventually widely introduced in the 1970s to restrict exposure to asbestos with the use of protective respirators and exhaust ventilation, and the substitution of other materials where possible. However, the long lag interval between the inhalation of asbestos and the development of disease means that asbestos-related lung disease is still all too common. It is important to have a clear understanding of the different diseases related to asbestos exposure (Fig. 15.4) as they each have very different manifestations and prognosis.

• *Asbestosis*: asbestosis is a pneumoconiosis in which **diffuse parenchymal lung fibrosis** develops as a result of heavy prolonged exposure to asbestos. The lag interval between exposure and the onset of the disease is typically 10–25 years, and is shorter the more intense the exposure. The clinical features are similar to those of other interstitial lung diseases such as cryptogenic fibrosing alveolitis, with **cough**, progressive **dyspnoea**, bibasal **crackles**, frequently **clubbing**, and a **restrictive ventilatory defect** (reduced lung volumes) with **impaired gas diffusion** (reduced transfer factor for carbon monoxide). Chest X-ray shows bilateral **reticulonodular shadowing**. Computed tomography

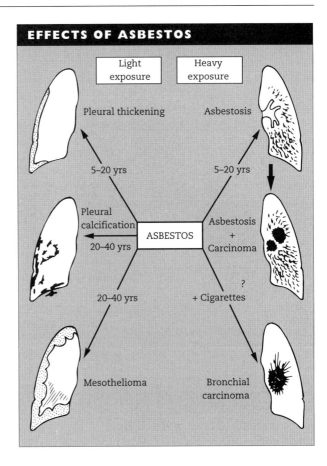

Fig. 15.4 Pulmonary diseases relating to exposure to asbestos.

(CT) is more sensitive in detecting early changes. Fibrosis is usually first evident around the respiratory bronchioles at the lung bases, becoming more diffuse as the disease progresses. **Asbestos bodies**, consisting of an asbestos fibre coated with an iron-containing protein, are usually seen within areas of fibrosis on light or electron microscopy. The disease is usually slowly progressive even after exposure has ceased, and is not usually responsive to corticosteroids. Patients with asbestosis are at substantial risk of developing lung cancer. It seems likely that some individuals have an increased susceptibility to developing asbestosis, although the nature of this susceptibility is unknown.

• *Pleural plaques*: pleural plaques are often visible as an incidental finding on chest X-rays

of workers who have been exposed to asbestos. They are often calcified and appear as **dense white lines** on the pleura of the chest wall, diaphragm, pericardium and mediastinum. When seen face-on they form an irregular **'holly leaf' pattern** (Fig. 15.5). They consist of white fibrous tissue usually situated on the parietal pleura. They **do not give rise to any impairment** of lung function or disability.

• *Acute asbestos pleurisy and pleural effusions*: many years after first exposure to asbestos, patients may develop episodes of pleurisy with **pleuritic pain** and **pleural effusions**. The pleural fluid is an **exudate** which is often **bloodstained** even in the absence of malignancy. There is sometimes associated elevation of erythrocyte sedimentation rate (ESR). Other causes of pleural effusion need to be

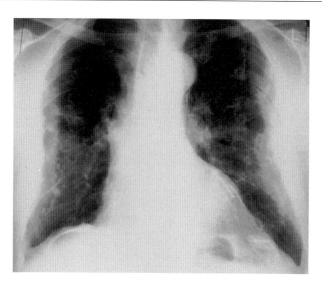

Fig. 15.5 This 70-year-old man had had extensive exposure to asbestos when he worked as a pipe lagger in shipyards. His chest X-ray shows extensive calcified pleural plaques seen as dense white lines over the diaphragm and pericardium, and demonstrating a 'holly leaf' pattern when seen face-on over the mid zones of the lungs. There is pleural thickening in both mid zones with some blunting of the costophrenic angles.

excluded. Pleural biopsy only shows evidence of inflammation and fibrosis without any specific diagnostic features. There is usually spontaneous resolution but recurrent episodes affecting both sides may occur and may lead to pleural thickening.

• *Pleural thickening*: localized or diffuse thickening and fibrosis of the pleura may develop as a result of asbestos exposure. There may be a history of recurrent episodes of acute pleurisy although these are often subclinical. The pleural thickening is usually most marked at the lung bases with **obliteration of the costophrenic angles**. It may initially be unilateral but often becomes bilateral. Areas of fibrous strands extending from the thickened pleura may give the appearance of **'crows feet'** on X-ray and **rolled atelectasis** may appear as a rounded opacity caused by puckering of the lung by the thickened pleura. When the pleural thickening is extensive it causes **dyspnoea** and a **restrictive ventilatory defect**.

• *Asbestos-related lung cancer*: epidemiology studies show an increased risk of lung cancer in workers in the asbestos industry with an approximately linear relationship between the dose of asbestos and the occurrence of lung cancer. The interaction between **asbestos** and **smoking** is multiplicative. The clinical features, distribution of cell type, investigation and treatment of asbestos-related lung cancers are the same as for those not associated with asbestos exposure (see Chapter 13) but impairment of lung function due to asbestosis may preclude surgery. At present, in the UK, workers are entitled to compensation from the Department of Social Security for asbestos-related lung cancer only if it occurs in association with asbestosis or diffuse pleural thickening.

• *Mesothelioma* is a **malignant tumour of the pleura** which is associated with a history of asbestos exposure in at least 90% of cases. The risk is greatest in those exposed to **crocidolite (blue asbestos)**. Sometimes the period of exposure to asbestos may have been as short as a few months. At present there are about 1000 deaths each year in the UK from mesothelioma and the incidence is expected to continue to rise until about the year 2010 since effective controls on asbestos exposure were only widely introduced in the 1970s and there is an average **lag interval of 20–40 years** between exposure to asbestos and the development of mesothelioma. It usually presents with **pain, dyspnoea, weight loss** and **lethargy**, and features of a **pleural effusion** sometimes associated with a lobulated pleural mass on X-ray. As the tumour progresses it encases the lung and may involve the pericardium and peritoneum, and give rise to blood-borne metastases. Histopathological diagnosis can be difficult to establish and biopsy procedures may not be warranted in cases with characteristic clinical and radiological features. Pleural fluid cytology and histology of percutaneous or thoracoscopic pleural biopsies should be interpreted in conjunction with the full clinical details as it can be difficult to distinguish between reactive and malignant mesothelial changes, and between secondary adenocarcinoma of the pleura and mesothelioma. The tumour has a tendency to spread along needle biopsy tracks giving rise to cutaneous nodules. Local radiotherapy is therefore often given to the site of biopsy to reduce this risk. Prognosis is poor, with most patients **dying within 2 years** of diagnosis. Unfortu-nately there is no effective treatment and management focuses on **palliation of symptoms** (e.g. high-dose opiate analgesia) and support of the patient.

Patients who have suffered disability as a result of occupational lung disease have a statutory right to receive **compensation** from governmental agencies such as the Department of Social Security in the UK. In some cases they may wish to pursue **litigation** against their employer. The death of a patient with a suspected occupational lung disease should be reported to the relevant authority, such as the **coroner**, who may wish to undertake a **post-mortem examination**.

Further reading

Cartier A. Definition and diagnosis of occupational asthma. *Eur Respir J* 1994; **7**: 153–60.

Craighead JE, Mossman BT. The pathogenesis of asbestos-associated diseases. *N Engl J Med* 1982; **306**: 1446–55.

Edge JR. Mesothelioma. *Br J Hosp Med* 1983; **29**: 521–36.

Hendrick DJ. Management of occupational asthma. *Eur Respir J* 1994; **7**: 961–8.

McLaren W, Soutar CA. Progressive massive fibrosis and simple pneumoconiosis in ex-miners. *Br J Ind Med* 1985; **42**: 734–40.

CHAPTER 16

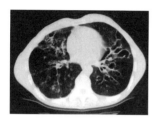

Pulmonary Vascular Disease

Pulmonary embolism

It is estimated that pulmonary emboli occur in about 1% of patients admitted to hospital and are directly responsible for about 5% of all deaths in hospital. The thrombus typically lurks silently in the deep veins of the legs of patients on surgical, medical and obstetric wards like a treacherous assassin lying in wait to claim the life of the victim by suddenly shooting off a major embolus to the lungs. Strategies to defend against this killer rely on widespread use of subcutaneous heparin prophylaxis against deep vein thrombosis (DVT) and rapid resort to full anti-coagulation (e.g. intravenous heparin) pending definitive investigations, in patients showing features suggesting DVT or a non-fatal pulmonary embolism.

Deep vein thrombosis

Factors predisposing to venous thrombosis were described by Virchow as a triad of venous stasis, damage to the wall of the vein and hypercoagulable states.

- *Venous stasis* occurs due to **immobility** (e.g. bed-bound patients, prolonged surgery, aeroplane flights), **local pressure** (e.g. tight plaster of Paris), **venous obstruction** (e.g. pressure of a pelvic tumour, pregnancy, obesity, varicose veins), congestive **cardiac failure** and **dehydration**.
- *Damage to a vein* occurs from local **trauma** to the vein, **previous thrombosis** and **inflammation** (phlebitis).
- *Hypercoagulable* states arise as part of the body's response to **surgery**, **trauma** and **childbirth**, and are found in association with **malignancy** and use of **oral contraceptives**. Recurrent thrombosis is particularly likely to occur where there are specific abnormalities of the clotting system such as **factor V Leiden, anti-thrombin III, protein S** or **protein C deficiencies** and in **anti-cardiolipin antibody** disease. Patients with recurrent or unexplained thromboembolic disease should have specific tests for these conditions since long-term anti-coagulation is advisable.

Pulmonary embolism is particularly common when thrombosis occurs in the proximal femoral or iliac veins and is less likely to occur when thrombosis is confined to the calf veins. Most pulmonary emboli arise in the deep veins of the legs but they may occasionally arise from thrombus in the inferior vena cava, the right side of the heart or from indwelling catheters in the subclavian or jugular veins. DVT may cause permanent damage to the vein with impairment of venous drainage, oedema, pigmentation, ulceration and an increased risk of further thrombosis.

The classic signs of DVT are oedema of the leg with tenderness, erythema and pain on flexing the ankle (Homan's sign). However, thrombosis in the deep veins of the leg, pelvis or abdomen may be completely silent. Available investigations for detecting DVT include **venography** whereby injection of radiocontrast material outlines thrombus, **ultrasound techniques** (e.g. compression ultrasound and colour flow Doppler), and **^{125}I-fibrinogen isotope scan** which demonstrates incorporation of radiolabelled fibrinogen into the thrombus.

Clinical features

The clinical features of pulmonary embolism depend upon the size and severity of the embolism, as summarized in Fig. 16.1, although there is overlap between the different presentations. In **acute massive pulmonary embolism** the picture is often that of a patient recovering from recent surgery who collapses. Attempts at resuscitation are often unsuccessful and there is a rapid high mortality, with very limited opportunity for intervention. Occlusion of a large part of the pulmonary circulation produces a catastrophic drop in cardiac output and the patient collapses with hypotension, cyanosis, tachypnoea and engorged neck veins. Sometimes the presentation is more **subacute**, as a series of emboli progressively occlude the pulmonary circulation over a longer period of time, with the patient developing progressive dyspnoea, tachypnoea and hypoxaemia. **Acute minor pulmonary embolism** presents as dyspnoea, typically accompanied by pleuritic pain, haemoptysis and fever if there is associated **pulmonary infarction**. Prompt recognition and treatment of an acute minor embolism may prevent the occurrence of a massive embolism. **Chronic thromboembolic pulmonary hypertension** is an unusual condition in which recurrent emboli progressively occlude the pulmonary circulation giving rise to progressive dyspnoea, pulmonary hypertension and right heart failure.

Investigation

General investigations

General investigations may yield clues that point towards a diagnosis of pulmonary embolism and are particularly useful in excluding alternative diagnoses.

• *Chest X-ray* is often normal but **elevation of a hemidiaphragm** and areas of **linear atelectasis** are suggestive of pulmonary emboli. A small **pleural effusion** with **wedge-shaped peripheral opacities** may occur in association with pulmonary infarction, and rarely an area of lung infarction undergoes cavitation. In massive embolism an **area of underperfusion** with few vascular markings may be apparent. **Enlarged pulmonary** arteries are a feature of pulmonary hypertension in chronic thromboembolic disease. The chest X-ray helps exclude alternative diagnoses such as pneumothorax, pneumonia and pulmonary oedema.

• *Electrocardiogram* is often normal apart from showing a **sinus tachycardia**. In major pulmonary embolism there may be features of **right heart strain** with depression of the ST segment and T wave in leads V_1–V_3, and evidence of right axis deviation with an $S_1 Q_3 T_3$ pattern. The electrocardiogram (ECG) helps exclude myocardial infarction and cardiac arrhythmias.

• *Arterial blood gases*: characteristically pulmonary embolism is associated with ventilation of underperfused areas of lung resulting in hypoxaemia and hyperventilation so that arterial blood gases show a reduced P_{O_2} and P_{CO_2}.

• *Lung function tests* are not usually helpful in the acute situation but in patients with dyspnoea due to chronic or subacute pulmonary emboli there is reduced gas diffusion with a reduction in the transfer factor for carbon monoxide. Lung function tests may also help identify other lung diseases (e.g. chronic obstructive pulmonary disease (COPD) and emphysema).

• *Blood tests*: there may be evidence of intravascular thrombosis (thrombin–antithrombin III complex assay) and fibrinolysis (fibrin degradation products). D-dimer is a breakdown product of crosslinked fibrin and levels are elevated in patients with thromboembolism. Levels, however, are also often elevated in other hospitalized patients so that

PULMONARY EMBOLISM

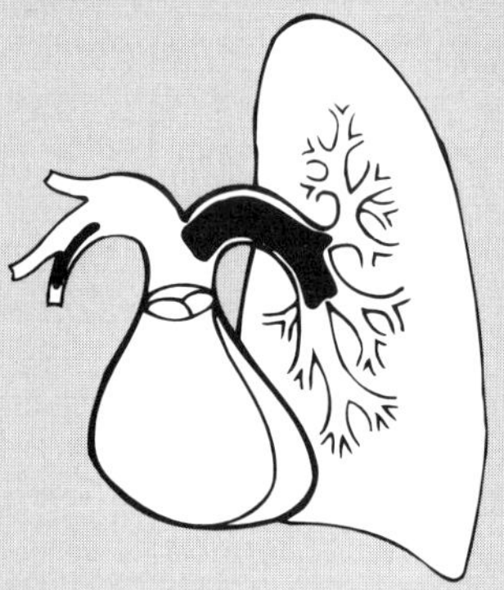

(a)

Massive pulmonary embolism

Acute

> 50% occlusion of circulation

Sudden circulatory collapse. Cyanosis

Central chest pain

Hyperventilation. Engorged neck veins

ECG: sometimes S1, Q3, T3 pattern

CXR: usually unhelpful

Angiography: shows filling defects and poor perfusion

Scan: usually not done

Subacute

> 50% occlusion of circulation

Progressive severe dyspnoea over few weeks without
obvious cause. Dyspnoea even at rest

Raised jugular vein pulse, sometimes loud P2

ECG: may show right ventricular hypertrophy (RVH)

CXR: may show infarcts

Angiography and scan: always severe perfusion defects

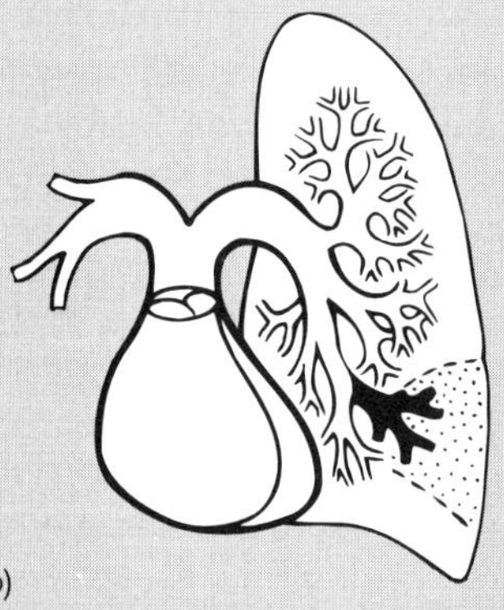

(b)

Acute minor pulmonary embolism

With infarction

Pleural pain haemoptysis, effusion, fever, hyperventilation

CXR: segmental collapse/consolidation

Without infarction

May be 'silent'

? Dyspnoea, hyperventilation

? Fever

CXR: may be normal

ECG: unhelpful

Angiography: usually shows obstruction if early

Scan: shows perfusion defects

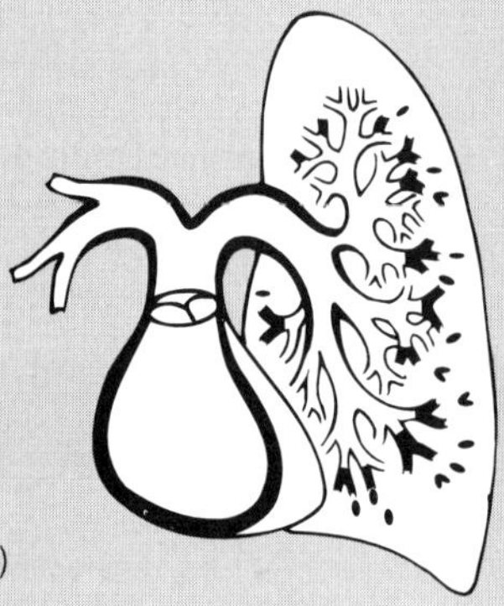

(c)

Chronic thromboembolic pulmonary hypertension

(repeated small emboli)

Progressive breathlessness, hyperventilation

? Effort syncope

Clinical features of pulmonary hypertension

ECG: right ventricular hypertrophy and axis deviation

CXR: prominent pulmonary artery

Angiography: may be normal or show slow circulation
or peripheral 'pruning'

Scan: expected to show patchy irregularity of perfusion.

Fig. 16.1 Synopsis of pulmonary embolism.

CHEST X-RAY AND V/Q SCAN

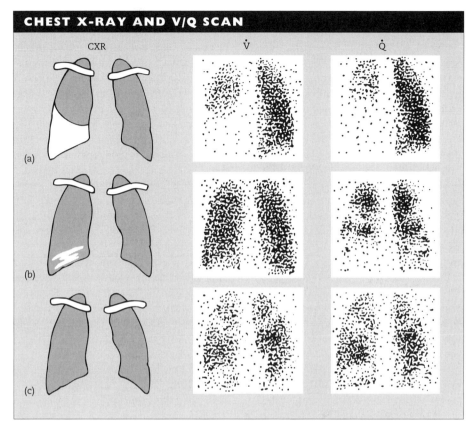

Fig. 16.2 Diagrammatic representation of the chest X-ray (CXR) appearances, together with ventilation ($\dot{V}$) and perfusion ($\dot{Q}$) images obtained with a gamma camera in three patients. Only anterior projections are shown. In practice posterior, lateral and oblique projections would be obtained for perfusion images (and, less commonly, ventilation images). In the diagram, ventilation images are shown at a stage before complete equilibrium is established.

(a) *Large right pleural effusion.* Ventilation is reduced on the right as expected. Perfusion is also reduced as expected. Even though perfusion seems proportionately more reduced than ventilation, the diversion of blood flow is in keeping with that commonly seen in pleural effusion and the overall distribution of perfusion resembles that of ventilation—there is a 'matching defect'.

(b) *Pulmonary embolism.* In this particular case, the chest X-ray shows only trivial changes at the right base. Ventilation is uniformly distributed but there are several major defects in the distribution of perfusion. These are 'non-matching defects'. Such defects are typical of pulmonary embolism and the appearances shown are diagnostic of multiple pulmonary embolism. Radiological shadowing in the lung fields, of whatever cause, is almost inevitably accompanied by abnormality of ventilation and/or perfusion at that site. The interest as in case (b), then centres on the other radiologically normal areas of lung.

(c) *Severe airways obstruction.* It is common for quite marked regional defects of ventilation and perfusion to accompany severe airways obstruction. The chest X-ray may show only overinflation. Usually the distribution of perfusion and that of ventilation are broadly similar (matching defects) as in (c).

D-dimer assays can be used to exclude, but not to confirm venous thromboembolism.

Specific investigations

• *Pulmonary angiography* is the definitive test for diagnosing pulmonary embolism but it is an invasive test requiring specialist expertise and equipment which are not widely available, and it is associated with a small risk, particularly in critically ill patients. A catheter is passed from a peripheral vein (e.g. femoral vein), through the right side of the heart into the pulmonary arteries, and radiocontrast material is injected and a rapid sequence of X-rays is taken. The angiographic features of embolism are intraluminal filling defects, abrupt cut off of vessels, peripheral pruning of vessels and areas of reduced perfusion.

• *Ventilation/perfusion (V/Q) lung scan* (Fig. 16.2): macroaggregrated particles or microspheres of human albumin, labelled with a gamma-emitting radioisotope, technetium-99m, are injected intravenously. These particles impact in the pulmonary capillaries and the radioactivity emitted from the lung fields is detected by a gamma camera, thus outlining the distribution of pulmonary perfusion. The distribution of ventilation in the lungs is similarly outlined after the patient has inhaled radiolabelled xenon. A completely normal pattern of pulmonary perfusion is strong evidence against pulmonary embolism. 'Cold areas' are evident on the scan where there is defective blood flow and these may occur in association with localized abnormalities apparent on a chest X-ray (e.g. pleural effusion, carcinoma, bulla). In these circumstances ventilation is usually decreased in the same areas resulting in 'matched defects' in ventilation and perfusion scans. The classic pattern seen in pulmonary embolism consists of multiple areas of perfusion defects which are not matched with defects in ventilation. A V/Q scan may therefore show normal perfusion, in which case pulmonary embolism is unlikely ('**low probability**'), areas of perfusion defects not matched with ventilation defects in the presence of a normal chest X-ray which indicates a '**high probability**' of pulmonary embolism, or it may show matched ventilation and perfusion defects in which case interpretation is difficult and the scan is regarded as '**indeterminate**'. Patients with a suspected pulmonary embolism but an indeterminate scan require further imaging.

• *Computed tomography (CT) angiography* (Fig. 16.3): some modern CT scanners have the capacity to perform very rapid spiral images and this imaging technique combined with injection of a radiocontrast material into a peripheral vein can be used to identify large emboli in the central pulmonary arteries, although it may fail to detect smaller emboli in peripheral vessels.

• *Imaging of peripheral veins*: demonstration of thrombus in the peripheral veins by venography, Doppler ultrasound or ^{125}I-fibrinogen isotope scan provides support for the decision to anti-coagulate a patient who has clinical features of pulmonary embolism but an 'indeterminate' V/Q scan.

Treatment
Anti-coagulant therapy

When a clinical diagnosis of suspected pulmonary embolism or DVT has been made, anti-coagulants should be started at once unless there is a strong contraindication (e.g. active haemorrhage). The decision as to whether anti-coagulants should be continued in the long term is made later based upon subsequent investigations. Usually an **intravenous loading dose** of **5000 units of heparin** is given as a bolus and this is followed by a **continuous infusion** of 1000–2000 units/h ($\approx$ 15–25 units/kg/h). The activated partial thromboplastin time (APPT) is measured 6 hours later and the dose is adjusted to maintain the APPT at 1.5–2.5 times the control value. In DVT and non-life threatening pulmonary embolism, high-dose, low-molecular-weight heparin given subcutaneously (e.g. dalteparin 200 units/kg/day) achieves predictable, rapid anti-coagulation without the need for laboratory monitoring. Side-effects of heparin include haemorrhage, bruising and

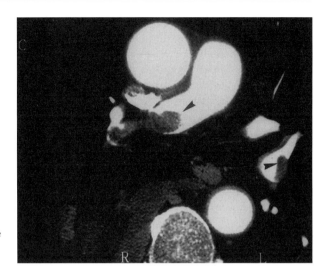

Fig. 16.3 Computed tomography (CT) pulmonary angiogram showing clot in the main pulmonary artery of the right lung (upper arrow) and the lower lobe pulmonary artery of the left lung (lower arrow).

thrombocytopenia. Once the clinical suspicion of pulmonary embolism or DVT has been supported by subsequent clinical circumstances or investigations (e.g. V/Q scan) **oral anticoagulation** is commenced using **warfarin**. Usually 10 mg are given on the first and second day as a loading dose, and then the INR (international normalized ratio) is measured and the dose adjusted to maintain a ratio of about 1.5–3.0. Warfarin takes at least 48–72 hours to establish its anti-coagulant effect so that heparin needs to be continued for this period. The optimal duration of warfarin treatment is uncertain but it is usually continued for 6 weeks to 3 months after a first episode of DVT or pulmonary embolism where this has occurred in association with a recognized risk factor (e.g. post-surgery, immobility, etc.). Patients with recurrent or unexplained thromboembolic disease should have investigations for hypercoagulable states performed (e.g. anti-thrombin III, protein S or C, deficiencies; anti-cardiolipin antibody disease) and may require indefinite anti-coagulation.

The patient should be given an **anticoagulant information booklet** which explains the nature and side-effects of treatment, states the indication for and proposed duration of treatment, contact numbers for obtaining advice, and instructions on avoiding medications which interfere with therapy. Many drugs enhance the effect of warfarin (e.g. non-steroidal anti-inflammatory drugs, aspirin, ciprofloxacin, erythromycin, etc.) and others reduce the effect (e.g. carbamazepine, barbiturates, rifampicin, etc.). Warfarin is teratogenic and women of child-bearing age should be warned of this danger, and may require specialist contraceptive advice. Precise details of INR, warfarin dosage and clinic appointments are included in the booklet which provides a useful method of communication with the patient and with all involved in the care of the patient (e.g. GP, dentist, nurses, etc.).

Thrombolytic therapy
The aim of thrombolytic therapy is to actively dissolve clot, but its use is reserved mainly for those patients with acute massive pulmonary embolism who remain in severe haemodynamic collapse (e.g. hypotensive, poorly perfused, hypoxaemic). These patients have survived the immediate impact of the pulmonary embolism but remain critically ill. If all the clinical features and bedside tests (e.g. ECG, chest X-ray) suggest a massive pulmonary embolism and exclude alternative diagnoses (pneumothorax, post-operative

haemorrhage, etc.), a decision may have to be taken that the circumstances justify the use of thrombolytic therapy. In some circumstances it may be possible to perform emergency angiography, and surgical embolectomy is occasionally possible where the patient is already in a cardiothoracic surgical unit, but thrombolytic therapy administered via a peripheral vein is probably equally effective. Contraindications to thrombolytic therapy include active haemorrhage, recent major surgery or trauma. Typically **streptokinase** 250 000 units is infused over 20 minutes, followed by 100 000 units/h for 24 hours. Thereafter heparin anticoagulation is commenced. Hydrocortisone 100 mg is given with the streptokinase to reduce the frequency of side-effects such as anaphylaxis. Alternative thrombolytic agents include **urokinase** and **recombinant tissue plasminogen activator** (rtPA).

Patients with acute pulmonary embolism require **high-flow oxygen** to correct hypoxaemia, and **analgesia** (e.g. diamorphine) to relieve pain and distress. In patients with active haemorrhage contraindicating the use of anticoagulants **a venous interruption** procedure may be useful. This involves the passing of a specially designed filter into the inferior vena cava to prevent further emboli from reaching the lungs from DVT in the pelvis or lower limbs.

Deep vein thrombosis prophylaxis

A variety of measures are directed against Virchow's triad of factors predisposing to DVT. Early **ambulation**, use of graded elastic **compression stockings** and leg **exercises** reduce venous stasis. Prophylactic **low-dose heparin** is now widely used to reduce the risk for patients on surgical, obstetric and medical wards. Typically heparin 5000 units is given subcutaneously twice daily. Low-molecular-weight heparins (e.g. dalteparin) have a longer duration of action and may be more effective so that they are often given to high-risk patients (e.g. after hip replacement surgery) as dalteparin 2500–5000 units subcutaneously once daily.

Other materials which may occasionally embolize to the lungs include **fat** (after fracture of long bones), **amniotic fluid** (postpartum), **air** (e.g. from disconnected central venous lines), **tumour** (from tumour invasion of venous system), **infected vegetations** (from tricuspid endocarditis) and **foreign materials** (from contamination of drugs injected by drug misusers).

Pulmonary hypertension

In normal lungs the pulmonary arterial pressure is about 20/8 mmHg (compared with typical systemic artery systolic/diastolic pressures of 120/80 mmHg) and the mean pulmonary artery pressure is 12–15 mmHg. Pulmonary hypertension is a condition characterized by sustained elevation of pulmonary artery pressure and this usually occurs **secondary** to chronic lung disease, when it is often referred to as **cor pulmonale**, but in some cases there is no demonstrable cause and this is termed **primary pulmonary hypertension**.

Cor pulmonale

Some confusion arises from the differing ways in which this term is used but it essentially refers to the development of pulmonary hypertension and right ventricular hypertrophy secondary to disease of the lungs. **Hypoxaemia** is a powerful stimulus for pulmonary vasoconstriction and this is the most common mechanism giving rise to cor pulmonale (e.g. chronic hypercapnic respiratory failure in COPD). Other mechanisms giving rise to pulmonary hypertension include **vascular obstruction** (e.g. chronic pulmonary emboli, pulmonary artery stenosis), **increased blood flow** (e.g. left to right intracardiac shunts — atrial and ventricular septal defects) and **loss of pulmonary vascular bed** (e.g. fibrotic lung disease, emphysema).

The clinical features of cor pulmonale are **elevation of jugular venous pressure**, **hepatomegaly** (due to congestion) peripheral **oedema**, a prominent left **parasternal** heave, a **loud pulmonary secondary sound** and a systolic murmur of **tricuspid regurgitation**. A chest X-ray may show large pulmonary arteries with pruning of the vessels in the lung fields. ECG typically shows p pulmonale (tall p wave in leads II III AVF) with a tall R wave in V_1 and ST segment depression with T-wave inversion in V_1–V_3. Echocardiography can assess the structure and dimension of the right heart chambers and the pulmonary artery pressure can be estimated from the velocity of the tricuspid regurgitation jet.

Idiopathic primary pulmonary hypertension

This is a rare disease, affecting about 2 per million of the population, in which pulmonary hypertension occurs without a demonstrable cause. It particularly affects young women. A small number of cases are inherited as an autosomal dominant trait and some cases are associated with human immunodeficiency virus (HIV) infection or with use of appetite suppressant drugs (e.g. aminorex, fenfluramine) but in most cases no cause is apparent. Patients present with dyspnoea, fatigue, angina and syncope on exertion. Investigations (e.g. echocardiography, *V/Q* scans, pulmonary artery catheterization) are particularly directed towards excluding secondary causes of pulmonary hypertension such as left to right cardiac shunts and chronic thromboembolic disease. The pathophysiology of the disease involves pulmonary artery vasoconstriction, vascular wall remodelling and thrombosis *in situ*. Treatment involves vasodilators (e.g. oral nifedipine, intravenous prostacycline infused continuously via a central venous cannula) and anti-coagulants, but heart–lung or lung transplantation need to be considered as the disease is usually relentlessly progressive.

Pulmonary vasculitis

When pulmonary vasculitis occurs it is usually as part of a more widespread systemic vasculitis such as Wegener's granulomatosis, polyarteritis nodosa, Churg–Strauss syndrome, Goodpasture's disease or collagen vascular diseases (e.g. scleroderma, systemic lupus erythematosus: see also Chapter 14).

Wegener's granulomatosis

This is characterized by necrotizing granulomatous inflammation and vasculitis affecting in particular the **upper airways** (rhinitis, sinusitis, bloodstained nasal discharge), the **lungs** (cavitating nodules, endobronchial disease) and **kidneys** (glomerulonephritis). **Antineutrophil cytoplasmic antibodies** (ANCA) are usually present in the serum. It is treated with a combination of corticosteroids and cyclophosphamide.

Churg–Strauss syndrome

This is an unusual disease consisting of allergic granulomatosis and angiitis. It consists of an initial phase of **asthma** followed by marked peripheral blood **eosinophilia** and **eosinophilic vasculitis** giving rise to pulmonary infiltrates, myocarditis, myositis, neuritis, rashes and glomerulonephritis. It usually responds rapidly to corticosteroids.

Polyarteritis nodosa

This consists of a vasculitis of medium and small arteries resulting in **aneurysm** formation, **glomerulonephritis** and **vasculitic lesions** in various organs. Pulmonary involvement is unusual but may result in haemoptysis, pulmonary haemorrhage, fibrosis and pleurisy. There is often considerable overlap in the clinical features of the various vasculitic syndromes.

Goodpasture's syndrome

This consists of a combination of **glomerulonephritis** and **alveolar haemorrhage** in association with circulating **anti-basement membrane antibody** which binds to lung and renal tissue. Pulmonary involvement is more common in smokers and may cause severe pulmonary haemorrhage resulting in haemoptysis, infiltrates on chest X-ray, hypoxaemia and anaemia. Transfer factor may be elevated due to binding of the inhaled carbon monoxide to haemoglobin in the alveoli. Treatment consists of corticosteroids and cyclophosphamide, with plasmapheresis to remove circulating antibodies.

Further reading

Burns A. Pulmonary vasculitis. *Br J Hosp Med* 1997; **58**: 389–92.

Corris P, Ellis D, Foley N, Miller A. Suspected acute pulmonary embolism: a practical approach. *Thorax* 1997; **52** (Suppl. 4): 1–24.

Ginsberg JS. Management of venous thromboembolism. *N Engl J Med* 1996; **335**: 1816–27.

Rubin LJ. Primary pulmonary hypertension. *N Engl J Med* 1997; **336**: 111–17.

Stein PD, Henry JW. Prevalence of acute pulmonary embolism among patients in a general hospital and at autopsy. *Chest* 1995; **108**: 978–81.

CHAPTER 17

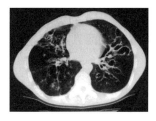

Pneumothorax and Pleural Effusion

Pneumothorax

Pneumothorax is the presence of air in the pleural space. Usually the air enters the pleural space as the result of a leak from a hole in the underlying lung but rarely it enters from outside as a result of chest injury. Pneumothoraces may be classified as **spontaneous** or **traumatic**, and spontaneous pneumothoraces may be **primary**, without evidence of other lung disease, or occur **secondary** to underlying lung disease (e.g. chronic obstructive pulmonary disease (COPD)).

Pathogenesis

Spontaneous primary pneumothorax typically occurs in a previously healthy young adult and is most common in tall thin men. Most seem to arise from the rupture of **subpleural blebs or bullae** at the apex of an otherwise normal lung. The aetiology of these blebs is uncertain but they may represent congenital lesions aggravated by the more negative pleural space pressure at the apex of the lung. Smoking increases the risk of a first spontaneous pneumothorax by approximately ninefold in women and twenty-twofold in men. The intrapleural pressure is normally negative due to the retractive force of lung elastic recoil so that when a communication is established between the atmosphere and the pleural space air is sucked in and the lung deflates. A small hole in the lung often closes off as the lung deflates.

Sometimes the hole remains open and the air leak will then continue until the pressure equalizes. Occasionally the opening from the lung to the pleural space functions as a valve allowing air to leak into the pleural space during inspiration but not to re-enter the lung on expiration. This is a potentially lethal situation as the air accumulates in the pleural space under increasing pressure giving a **tension pneumothorax** in which the lung is pushed down, the mediastinum is shifted to the opposite side and the venous return to the heart and cardiac output are impaired.

There is an increased risk of pneumothorax in association with virtually all lung diseases. These spontaneous secondary pneumothoraces are particularly common in patients with COPD and bullous emphysema. A pneumothorax resulting from rupture of a bulla may render an already disabled patient critically ill. Pneumothorax is a well-recognized complication of positive pressure endotracheal ventilation on intensive therapy units (ITUs) of patients with underlying lung disease. Traumatic pneumothorax usually arises from puncture of the lung by a fractured rib but air may enter the pleural space from outside via a penetrating injury or from rupture of alveoli, oesophagus, trachea or bronchi. **Iatrogenic** ('doctor-induced') pneumothorax may arise as a complication of invasive chest procedures such as the insertion of a catheter into the subclavian vein, percutaneous needle aspiration of a lung lesion, or transbronchial lung biopsy.

Clinical features

Pneumothorax typically presents with acute **pleuritic pain** and **breathlessness**. An otherwise healthy young adult may tolerate a pneumothorax quite well but older patients with underlying lung disease often develop severe respiratory distress with cyanosis. The clinical signs of pneumothorax are **reduced breath sounds** and **hyper-resonance** on the side of the pneumothorax, but these may be difficult to detect. Sometimes a left-sided pneumothorax is associated with a clicking noise if the cardiac beat produces friction on movement of the layers of the pleura. Signs of **mediastinal shift** such as displacement of the trachea and apex beat to the opposite side may be detectable in a tension pneumothorax.

The **chest X-ray** shows a black gas space, containing no lung markings, between the margin of the collapsed lung and the chest wall (Fig. 17.1). A chest X-ray taken after expiration may be needed to detect a small pneumothorax. It is often difficult to detect a pneumothorax if the chest X-ray is performed with the patient lying supine (e.g. on ventilation in the ITU) since the air in the pleural space, in this position, rises anteriorly giving an appearance of hyperlucency of the lower chest. If the patient cannot be X-rayed

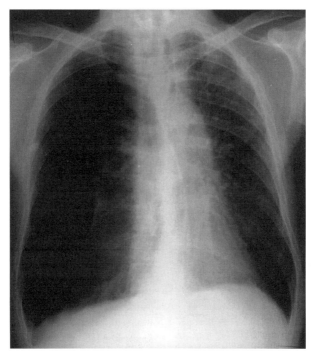

Fig. 17.1 This 55-year-old man with chronic perihilar fibrosis due to sarcoidosis developed acute dyspnoea and right pleuritic pain followed by increasing respiratory distress. On arrival in hospital examination showed diminished breath sounds and hyper-resonance over the right lung field, with deviation of the trachea to the left. Chest X-ray shows a right tension pneumothorax with a large gas-filled pleural space without lung markings in the right hemithorax, deflation of the right lung and shift of the mediastinum to the left. He was given oxygen and analgesia, and an intercostal chest tube was inserted into the right pleural space as an emergency procedure in the casualty department, with successful re-expansion of the lung and relief of his respiratory distress.

upright, a lateral decubitus film should be performed.

Treatment

• *No intervention*: a small (<20% of hemithorax) pneumothorax which is not causing respiratory distress may not require any intervention since it will **resolve spontaneously at a rate of about 1–2% per day**. Such patients may be allowed home with advice to return to hospital immediately if symptoms deteriorate. They should not undertake an aeroplane flight until the pneumothorax has resolved since the reduced barometric pressure at altitude causes expansion of enclosed thoracic air pockets. A follow-up appointment should be arranged for clinical assessment and chest X-ray to ensure resolution of the pneumothorax and to exclude underlying lung disease.

• *Aspiration*: air may be aspirated from the pleural space by inserting a French gauge 16 cannula (such as an intravenous cannula) through the second intercostal space in the mid-clavicular line after injection of local anaesthetic. Once the pleural cavity is entered, the needle is removed and the cannula is connected via a three-way tip to a syringe, and air is aspirated. A chest X-ray is performed to assess the success of the procedure. This technique is simple and less distressing to the patient than insertion of a chest tube. Even large pneumothoraces can be aspirated but chest tube insertion is needed if aspiration is unsuccessful, if there is a persistent air leak from the lung or if there is a tension pneumothorax.

• *Intercostal tube drainage* (Fig. 17.2): the insertion of a chest tube is a frightening procedure for the patient, who needs adequate **explanation and reassurance**. Pre-medication with atropine (300–600 μg IV) prevents vasovagal reactions, and a small dose of a sedative (e.g. midazolam 1–2 mg IV) may be helpful for very anxious patients. The chest X-ray should be studied to confirm the correct side and location for insertion of the tube. This is usually the fourth, fifth or sixth intercostal space in the

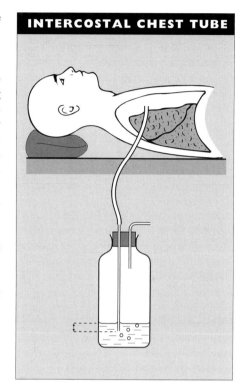

INTERCOSTAL CHEST TUBE

Fig. 17.2 Intercostal chest tube *in situ* connected to an underwater seal. The end of the tube is 2–3 cm below the level of the water in the bottle. Oscillation of the meniscus of the water in the tube on respiration indicates that the tube is patent. Bubbling on respiration or coughing indicates continued drainage of air.

mid-axillary line. Sterile gloves are worn and the skin is cleaned with antiseptic solution. The skin, subcutaneous tissues, intercostal muscles and parietal pleura are anaesthetized by injection of 10–20 ml of 1% **lignocaine**. Aspiration of air into the syringe confirms that the pleural space has been entered. The skin is incised and **blunt dissection** with a forceps is used to make a track through the intercostal muscles into the pleural space, taking care to avoid the neurovascular bundle situated in a groove on the lower surface of each rib. The chest drain (e.g. size 24 French gauge (Fr)) may then be inserted through the track, guided by a forceps or by a trocar which can be helpful in directing the tube towards the apex. The track made by blunt dissection should be sufficiently wide to **allow the drain to slide in easily without force**, and care must be taken to avoid causing damage to the underlying lung or other structures. The tube is then **connected to an underwater seal**, and is securely **anchored in place** with a strong suture. Breathing with a chest tube in place is painful and **adequate analgesia** should be prescribed. The position of the tube and the degree of re-expansion of the lung should be checked by chest X-ray.

Occasionally a size 24 Fr tube is not adequate to cope with a large leak and air tracks alongside the drain causing subcutaneous emphysema. This requires insertion of a second, larger tube. Low-pressure suction applied to the tube may expedite the removal of air. High-pressure suction may succeed in bringing the pleural surfaces into apposition thereby sealing off the leak.

• *Surgical intervention*: surgical treatment is required for persistent or recurrent pneumothoraces. Failure of re-expansion of the lung with profuse bubbling of air through the underwater drain suggests a bronchopleural fistula (i.e. a persistent communication between the lung and pleural space). **Surgical closure of the hole** with pleurodesis is usually necessary and may be performed via a thoracotomy or via thoracoscopy. The hole is oversewn and blebs on the surface of the lung are excised. **Pleurodesis** involves the obliteration of the pleural space and can be achieved by instilling tetracycline or talc which provokes adhesions between the visceral and parietal pleura. **Pleurectomy** involves the removal of the parietal pleural. Usually an apicolateral pleurectomy (leaving the posterobasal pleura intact) prevents recurrence without compromising lung function. There is a risk of recurrence of approximately 20% after a first spontaneous pneumothorax and a 50% risk after a second pneumothorax. Surgical intervention is therefore usually recommended after a second pneumothorax. This is also the case if the patient has suffered a pneumothorax on both sides, because of the risk of cata-

strophic simultaneous bilateral pneumothoraces. Particular thought must be given to the best procedure for young adults with complicated pneumothoraces secondary to diseases such as cystic fibrosis so as not to compromise potential future lung transplantion. A limited apicolateral surgical abrasion pleurodesis may be the best option in these circumstances.

Pleural effusion

A pleural effusion is a collection of fluid in the pleural space.

Pleural fluid dynamics

The parietal and visceral pleural surfaces are normally in close contact and the potential space between them contains only a very thin layer of fluid. Pleural fluid dynamics are complex and incompletely understood but Fig. 17.3 shows in a simplified form some of the main factors governing fluid filtration and absorption. The parietal pleura is perfused by the systemic circulation, and the high systemic capillary pressure, negative intrapleural pressure and pleural oncotic pressure overcome the plasma oncotic pressure resulting in fluid filtration into the pleural space. The visceral pleura is mainly perfused by the pulmonary circulation with its low pulmonary capillary pressure so that the balance of forces results in movement of fluid outward from the pleural space to the veins and lymphatics. The balance between **fluid filtration** by the parietal pleura and **fluid absorption** by the visceral pleura is such that fluid does not normally collect in the pleural space. Pleural effusions may develop from **increased capillary pressure** (e.g. left ventricular failure), **reduced plasma oncotic pressure** (e.g. hypoalbuminaemia), **increased capillary permeability** (e.g. disease of pleura) or **obstruction of lymphatic drainage** (e.g. carcinoma of lymphatics).

Clinical features

Patients with pleural effusions typically present with **dyspnoea**, sometimes with pleuritic pain,

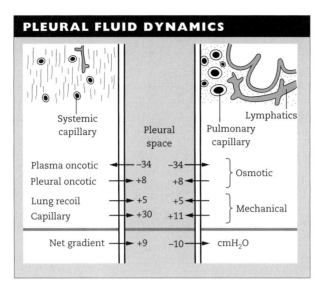

PLEURAL FLUID DYNAMICS

Fig. 17.3 Pleural fluid dynamics. In the normal pleural space the mechanical and oncotic pressures are in equilibrium such that net filtration of fluid by the parietal pleura is balanced by net absorption of fluid by the visceral pleura. Pleural effusion may arise from changes in the mechanical and oncotic pressures (transudates) or from increased capillary permeability due to disease of the pleura (exudates).

and often with features of associated diseases (e.g. cardiac failure, carcinoma, etc.). The signs of pleural effusion are **decreased expansion** on the side of the effusion, **stony dullness**, **diminished breath sounds** and **reduced tactile vocal fremitus**. Sometimes **bronchial breathing** is heard at the upper level of the fluid. In taking the patient's history it is important to enquire about clues to possible causes of pleural effusion such as asbestos exposure, contact with tuberculosis, smoking, drugs (e.g. dantrolene, bromocriptine) or systemic disease. A full careful physical examination is essential to detect signs of underlying disease (e.g. cardiac failure, breast lump, lymphadenopathy, etc.).

Investigations (Fig. 17.4)

• *Radiology*: **chest X-ray** characteristically shows a dense white shadow with a concave upper edge (Fig. 17.5). Small effusions cause no more than blunting of a costophrenic angle whereas very large effusions cause 'white out'

of an entire hemithorax with shift of the mediastinum to the opposite side. A **lateral decubitus** film may be useful in demonstrating mobility of the fluid, distinguishing the features from pleural thickening. **Ultrasound** imaging is helpful in localizing loculated effusions and in positioning chest tubes. **Computed tomography (CT)** may be required to assess the underlying lung and mediastinum.

• *Pleural fluid aspiration* is the key initial investigation. A **protein** level >30 g/L and **lactate dehydrogenase (LDH)** level >200 iu/L indicate that the effusion is an exudate and that further investigations for pleural disease are indicated. Both transudates and exudates are typically a yellow, straw colour. **Blood-stained** fluid points towards malignancy, pulmonary infarction or severe inflammation. **Pus** indicates an empyema, **milky** white fluid suggests a chylothorax and frank **blood** suggests a haemothorax (e.g. due to trauma). A low **glucose** content points towards infection or a connective tissue disease as a cause of the effu-

INVESTIGATION AND CAUSES OF PLEURAL EFFUSIONS

INVESTIGATION

Clinical features
Dyspnoea
Dull to percussion
↓Breath sounds
↓Tactile fremitus

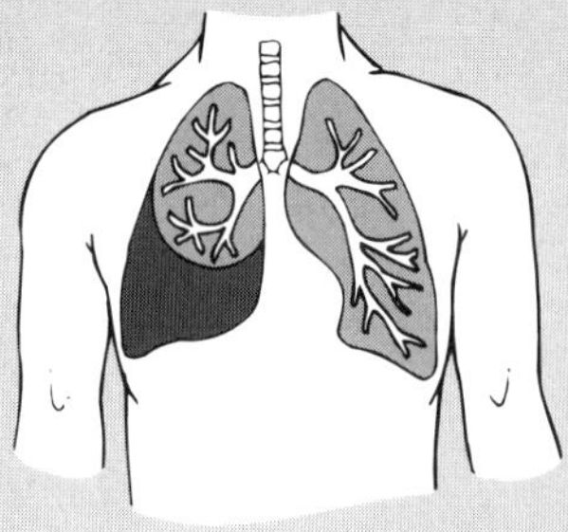

CLINICAL EXAMINATION

Pleural fluid aspiration
• APPEARANCE
Staw coloured
Bloodstained
Pus (empyema)
Blood (haemothorax)

• BIOCHEMISTRY
Protein > 30g/L (exudate)
LDH > 200 iu/L (exudate)
↑Amylase (pancreatitis)
↓Glucose (infection)

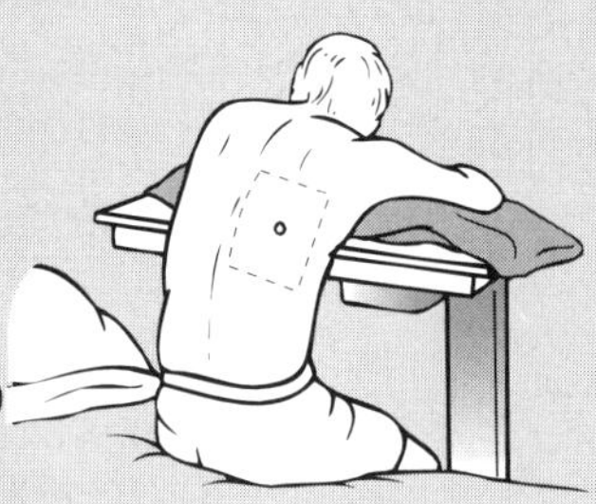

PLEURAL FLUID ASPIRATION

• CYTOLOGY
Lymphocytes (TB, tumour)
Neutrophils (infection,
   inflammation)
Malignant cells

• MICROBIOLOGY
TB, bacteria

Pleural biopsy
(Abram's needle; thoracoscopy)
• HISTOLOGY
Carcinoma, mesothelioma,
TB
• MICROBIOLOGY
TB

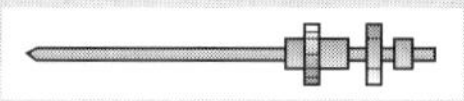

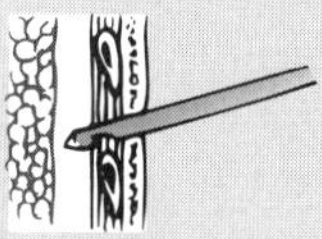

ABRAM'S NEEDLE BIOPSY

CAUSES

Transudates
(protein < 30g/L, LDH < 200 iu/L)
Cardiac failure
Renal failure
Hepatic cirrhosis
Ascites
Hypoproteinaemia
Myxoedema

Exudates
(protein > 30g/L, LDH > 200 iu/L)
• MALIGNANCY
Metastatic carcinoma
Mesothelioma
• INFECTION
TB
Parapneumonic
Empyema (pus)

• INFLAMMATION
SLE
Rheumatoid arthritis
Dressler's syndrome
Benign asbestos effusion
Drugs (e.g. dantrolene)

• SUBDIAPHRAGMATIC DISEASE
Subphrenic abscess
Ascites
Pancreatitis

Fig. 17.4 Summary of the causes and investigation and causes of pleural effusions.

sion. A high **amylase** content is characteristic of pleural effusion associated with pancreatitis but also sometimes occurs with adenocarcinoma. **Neutrophils** are the predominant cells in acute inflammation or infection and **lym-** **phocytes** in chronic effusions particularly due to tuberculosis or malignancy. **Cytology** may show malignant cells (e.g. mesothelioma or metastatic carcinoma). **Microbiology** examination of the fluid may identify tuberculosis or bacterial infection, for example.
• *Pleural biopsy* may be performed using a specially designed needle such as the **Abram's needle**. After injection of local anaesthetic,

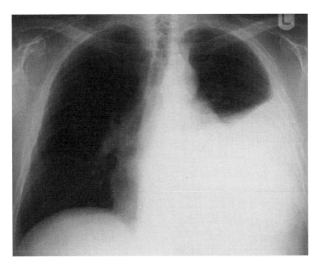

Fig. 17.5 This 68-year-old man presented with a 6-week history of progressive breathlessness and left pleuritic pain. On examination there was stony dullness and diminished breath sounds over the left hemithorax. The chest X-ray shows features of a large pleural effusion with a dense white shadow with a concave upper border over the left side of the chest. The pleural fluid was bloodstained and showed metastatic adenocarcinoma on cytology. Bronchoscopy showed the primary tumour partly occluding the left lower lobe bronchus. An intercostal drain was inserted to evacuate the fluid and tetracycline was instilled to achieve pleurodesis.

incision of the skin and blunt dissection of the intercostal muscles, the needle is passed into the pleural space. The Abram's needle is in two parts which can be rotated on each other: pleural fluid can be aspirated when the window of the needle is rotated to the open position. The needle is then pulled back until some parietal pleural tissue is caught in the notch of the needle. The inner cylinder of the needle has a sharp cutting edge which when rotated cuts off pleural tissue caught in the notch (Fig. 17.4). Histology of pleural biopsy samples is particularly useful in diagnosing malignant effusions or tuberculosis (e.g. caseating granuloma). A sample of the biopsy should also be sent for tuberculosis culture. **Video-assisted thoracoscopy**, which is usually performed under general anaesthesia, allows direct inspection of the pleural surfaces with direct biopsy of abnormal tissue.

Further investigations (e.g. bronchoscopy for suspected lung carcinoma or ultrasound of abdomen for suspected subphrenic disease) may be required depending on the clues to diagnosis elicited on initial assessment.

Causes

Pleural effusions are classified as transudates or exudates. Transudates are characterized by a low protein content (<30 g/L) and a low LDH level (<200 iu/L). They arise as a result of changes in hydrostatic or osmotic pressures across the pleural membrane rather than from disease of the pleura. Exudates are characterized by a high protein (>30 g/L) and LDH (>200 iu/L) content, and result from increased permeability associated with disease of the pleura. Sometimes in patients with borderline protein and LDH levels there is difficulty in distinguishing between transudates and exudates, and comparison of pleural to serum ratios may be helpful: exudates have a pleural fluid to serum protein ratio >0.5 and an LDH ratio >0.6.

Transudates

The main causes of transudative pleural effusions are **cardiac failure**, **renal failure**, **hepatic cirrhosis** and **hypoproteinaemia** due to malnutrition or nephrotic syndrome, for example. In most cases transudative effusions are bilateral, although they may be asymmetrical and initially unilateral. **Ascitic fluid** may pass through pleuroperitoneal communications, which are more common in the right hemidiaphragm. Similarly **peritoneal dialysis fluid** may give rise to a right pleural effusion. Rare causes of transudates are **myxoedema** and Meigs' syndrome (benign ovarian fibroma, ascites and pleural effusion, which may be a transudate or exudate). Sometimes treatment of cardiac failure with diuretics results in an increase in fluid protein content so that the effusion appears to be an exudate. Treatment of transudates involves correction of the underlying hydrostatic or osmotic mechanisms (e.g. treatment of cardiac failure or hypoproteinaemia), and further investigation of the pleura is not usually necessary.

Exudates

A variety of diseases which affect the pleura are associated with increased capillary permeability or reduced lymphatic drainage. Exudates are often unilateral and investigations are directed towards identifying the cause since this determines treatment.

• *Malignancy*: **metastases** to the pleura most commonly arise from **lung**, **breast**, **ovarian** or **gastrointestinal** cancers and from **lymphoma**. **Mesothelioma** is a primary tumour of the pleura related to asbestos exposure (see Chapter 15). In malignant effusions the fluid is often bloodstained with a high lymphocyte count, and cytology often shows malignant cells. If cytology of a pleural aspirate is negative, pleural biopsy may be diagnostic. Sometimes confirmation of the diagnosis is difficult and thoracoscopy with biopsy of lesions under direct vision may be necessary. Malignancy may give rise to pleural effusions by means other than direct involvement of the pleura.

Lymphatic involvement by tumours may obstruct drainage and cause pleural effusions with negative cytology. **Chylous effusions**, due to malignancy in the thoracic duct, are characterized by a milky cloudy appearance of the pleural fluid. **Superior vena caval obstruction** may give rise to pleural effusions due to elevation of systemic venous pressure. Treatment of a pleural effusion associated with malignancy is directed against the underlying tumour (e.g. chemotherapy). **Drainage of the fluid** by needle aspiration or intercostal chest tube relieves dyspnoea. It is usually advisable to remove the fluid slowly at no more than 1–1.5 litres at a time as too rapid removal may provoke re-expansion pulmonary oedema, although the risk is small. The risk of recurrence of the effusion may be reduced by intrapleural instillation of tetracycline (e.g. 1000 mg tetracycline in 40 ml saline with 10 ml of lignocaine, left *in situ* for 2 hours) to provoke **pleurodesis**. It is important that the effusion has been drained to dryness before insertion of tetracycline so that the two pleural surfaces can be apposed so as to promote adhesions. If tetracycline pleurodesis is not successful, surgical pleurodesis or **pleurectomy via thoracoscopy** may be helpful.

• *Infection*: pneumonia may be complicated by an inflammatory reaction in the pleura resulting in a **parapneumonic effusion**. Secondary infection of this effusion with multiplication of bacteria in the pleural space produces an **empyema** which is the presence of pus in the pleural cavity. If a parapneumonic effusion has a low pH (<7.1) there is a high risk of an empyema developing and early tube drainage is indicated. Various organisms may give rise to an empyema including *Streptococcus pneumoniae*, *Staphylococcus aureus*, *Streptococcus milleri* and anaerobic organisms (e.g. *Bacteroides*). Empyema is particularly associated with aspiration pneumonia (e.g. related to unconsciousness, alcohol, vomiting, dysphagia, etc.). **Actinomycosis** is an unusual infection which spreads from the lung to the pleura and chest wall with a tendency to form sinus tracts. **Tuberculosis** must always be borne in mind as a cause of pleural effusion or empyema (see Chapter 7).

Initial **antibiotic treatment** is often with amoxycillin and metronidazole, adjusted in accordance with results of microbiology tests. The key treatment of empyema, however, is **drainage of the pus**. Placement of the drainage tube is often best guided by ultrasound imaging as the effusion is often loculated due to fibrin deposition and adhesions. Instillation of a **fibrinolytic agent** (e.g. streptokinase 250 000 units in 20 ml of saline, left *in situ* for 2 hours, daily for 3–5 days) through the chest tube into the pleural space often improves drainage by promoting lysis of fibrin adhesions. **Surgical intervention** is necessary if these measures fail and a variety of approaches may be used including rib resection with open drainage, or thoracotomy with removal of infected debris and decortication (stripping of the pleura and empyematous sac).

• *Inflammatory diseases*: various inflammatory diseases may involve the pleura. Effusions associated with **connective tissue diseases** (e.g. rheumatoid arthritis, systemic lupus erythematosus) characteristically have a low glucose content. **Drug reactions** involving the pleura have been described with dantrolene, bromocriptine, nitrofurantoin and methlysergide, for example. **Asbestos** may give rise to **benign asbestos-related pleural effusions** which may recur producing diffuse pleural thickening (see Chapter 15). Small pleural effusions may complicate **pulmonary embolism** and infarction (see Chapter 16). **Dressler's syndrome** consists of inflammatory pericarditis and pleurisy of uncertain aetiology following a myocardial infarction or cardiac surgery.

• *Subdiaphragmatic disease*: **pancreatitis** may be associated with pleural effusions probably as a result of diaphragmatic inflammation. Such effusions are usually left sided and characterized by a high amylase content. **Ascites** may traverse the diaphragm through pleuroperitoneal communications causing a pleural effusion. Spread of infection or inflammation from a **subphrenic abscess** or **intrahepatic abscess** may also cause a pleural effusion.

Oesophageal rupture

Oesophageal rupture may give rise to a pyopneumothorax (air and pus in the pleural cavity). This may result from external **trauma** or be **iatrogenic** (e.g. perforation during endoscopy). **Spontaneous rupture of the oesophagus** (Boerhaave's syndrome) is a rare but catastrophic condition which typically occurs when the patient attempts to suppress vomiting by closure of the pharyngeal sphincter. Intra-oesophageal pressure rises steeply and rupture typically occurs in the lowest third of the oesophagus. It is a more severe form of the Mallory–Weiss syndrome of haematemesis due to mucosal tears from protracted vomiting. Characteristically vomiting is followed by chest pain and subcutaneous emphysema (palpable air in skin) as air and gastric contents leak into the mediastinum. A few hours later the pleural membrane gives way and air and food debris pass into the pleural cavity producing pleuritic pain, pleural effusion and empyema. Chest X-ray typically shows an initial pneumomediastinum (a rim of air around mediastinal structures) followed by a hydropneumothorax. The diagnosis is notoriously difficult to make and a radiocontrast oesophagogram is the key investigation. Thoracotomy with repair of the oesophagus is usually the best treatment.

Further reading

Dhillon DP, Spiro SG. Malignant pleural effusions. *Br J Hosp Med* 1983; **29**: 506–10.

Ferguson AD, Prescott RJ, Selkon JB, Watson D, Swinburn CR. The clinical course and management of thoracic empyema. *Q J Med* 1996; **89**: 285–9.

Hamm H, Light RW. Parapneumonic effusion and empyema. *Eur Respir J* 1997; **10**: 1150–6.

Miller AC, Harvey JE. Guidelines for the management of spontaneous pneumothorax. *BMJ* 1993; **307**: 114–16.

Miller KS, Sahan SA. Chest tubes: indications, technique, management and complications. *Chest* 1987; **91**: 258–64.

CHAPTER 18

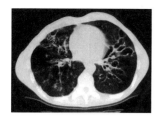

Acute Respiratory Distress Syndrome

Introduction

The acute respiratory distress syndrome (ARDS) is a form of **acute respiratory failure** due to **permeability pulmonary oedema** resulting from **endothelial damage** developing in response to an **initiating injury or illness**.

It had long been recognized that soldiers wounded in battle often died of respiratory failure some days later. During World Wars I and II it was thought that this was due to infection or excessive fluid administration. Further experience of the condition during the Vietnam War showed that despite successful surgical management of wounds and optimal fluid replacement soldiers were still dying of pulmonary dysfunction some days later and that the lungs showed features such as oedema, atelectasis, haemorrhage and hyaline membrane formation. It was not until 1967 that this condition was recognized as a specific clinical entity separate from the precipitating injury, and that it could also arise from civilian injuries and illnesses. The term adult respiratory distress syndrome was used because of the superficial similarity of the pathology of the disease, showing hyaline membranes, to the infant respiratory distress syndrome (due to surfactant deficiency in premature babies), although the term acute respiratory distress syndrome may be more appropriate.

Pathogenesis

In most situations pulmonary oedema arises as a result of increased pulmonary capillary **pressure** (e.g. left ventricular failure) but in ARDS it arises because of increased alveolar capillary **permeability**.

Pressure pulmonary oedema (Fig. 18.1)

In the normal situation the hydrostatic pressure and the osmotic pressure exerted by the plasma proteins are in a state of equilibrium between the pulmonary capillaries and lung alveoli. An **increase in hydrostatic pressure** is the commonest cause of pulmonary oedema and this typically occurs secondary to elevated left atrial pressure from left ventricular failure (e.g. after myocardial infarction) or from mitral valve disease (e.g. mitral stenosis). **Volume overload** may also increase pulmonary capillary pressure and this may arise from excessive intravenous fluid administration or fluid retention (e.g. renal failure). **Reduced osmotic pressure** may contribute to pulmonary oedema and this occurs in hypoproteinaemic states (e.g. severely ill, malnourished patients; nephrotic syndrome with renal protein loss). In the early stages of pulmonary oedema there is an increase in the fluid content of the interstitial space between the capillaries and alveoli but as the condition deteriorates flooding of the alveoli occurs.

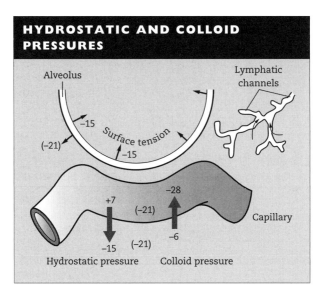

HYDROSTATIC AND COLLOID PRESSURES

Alveolus

Lymphatic channels

−15

(−21)

Surface tension

−15

−28

+7   (−21)

Capillary

−15   (−21)

−6

Hydrostatic pressure   Colloid pressure

Fig. 18.1 Diagram illustrating approximate values for hydrostatic and colloid pressures in millimetres of mercury (mmHg) between the pulmonary capillary and alveolus. Pulmonary oedema may arise from increased **hydrostatic** **pressure** (e.g. cardiogenic pulmonary oedema), from reduced **colloid pressure** (e.g. hypoalbuminaemia), or from increased capillary **permeability** (e.g. acute respiratory distress syndrome).

Permeability pulmonary oedema

In ARDS it is thought that a cascade of inflammatory events arises over a period of hours from a focus of tissue damage. In particular, activated neutrophils aggregate and adhere to endothelial cells, releasing various toxins, oxygen radicals and mediators (e.g. arachidonic acid, histamine, kinins). This complex process may be initiated by a variety of injuries or illnesses but the outcome is **endothelial damage** resulting in **increased alveolar capillary permeability**. The alveoli become filled with a protein-rich exudate containing abundant neutrophils and other inflammatory cells and the airspaces show a rim of proteinaceous material — the hyaline membrane. The characteristic feature of permeability pulmonary oedema in ARDS is that the pulmonary capillary wedge pressure is not elevated. This may be measured by passing a special balloon-tipped catheter (e.g. Swan–Ganz catheter) via a central vein through the right side of the heart to the pulmonary artery. The balloon of the catheter is then inflated and is carried forward in the blood flow until it wedges in a pulmonary capillary. The measurement of pulmonary capillary wedge pressure reflects left atrial pressure and in ARDS it is ≤18mmHg, whereas in cardiogenic pulmonary oedema it is elevated.

Clinical features

ARDS develops in response to a variety of injuries or illnesses which affect the lungs either **directly** (e.g. aspiration of gastric contents, severe pneumonia, lung contusion) or **indirectly** (e.g. systemic sepsis, major trauma, pancreatitis). About 12–48 hours after an initiating event the patient develops respiratory distress with increasing dyspnoea and tachypnoea. Arterial blood gases show deteriorating hypoxaemia which responds poorly to oxygen

INITIATING ILLNESSES OF ARDS	
Direct	**Indirect**
Aspiration of gastric contents	Sepsis
Severe pneumonia	Major trauma
Smoke inhalation	Multiple blood transfusions
Lung contusion	Pancreatitis
Fat embolism	Extensive burns
Amniotic fluid embolism	Anaphylaxis
Chemical inhalation (e.g. silo filler's lung)	Hypotensive shock
Oxygen toxicity/ventilator lung	Disseminated intravascular coagulation

Various illnesses and injuries, which affect the lungs directly or indirectly, initiate a cascade of inflammatory responses resulting in endothelial damage and the characteristic permeability pulmonary oedema of ARDS.

Table 18.1 Acute respiratory distress syndrome (ARDS): initiating injuries and illnesses.

therapy. Diffuse bilateral infiltrates develop on chest X-ray in the absence of evidence of cardiogenic pulmonary oedema. Although there is a spectrum of severity and ARDS evolves over a period of time, in full blown ARDS the characteristic features are as follows.

• A history of an **initiating injury or illness** (Table 18.1).

• **Hypoxaemia** refractory to oxygen therapy (e.g. $Po_2 < 8.0\,kPa$ (60 mmHg) on 40% oxygen). The degree of hypoxaemia may be expressed as the ratio of arterial oxygen tension (Po_2) to the fractional inspired oxygen concentration (F_iO_2: 100% oxygen = F_iO_2 of 1). In ARDS Po_2/F_iO_2 is < 26 kPa (200 mmHg).

• Bilateral diffuse infiltrates on chest X-ray (Fig. 18.2).

• No evidence of cardiogenic pulmonary oedema (e.g. **pulmonary capillary wedge pressure** ≤ 18 mmHg).

Treatment

The treatment of ARDS consists of optimal management of the initiating illness or injury combined with supportive care directed at preserving adequate oxygenation, maintaining optimal haemodynamic function and compensating for multi-organ failure which often supervenes.

Treatment of initiating illness

Prompt and complete treatment of the initiating injury or illness is essential. This includes rapid resuscitation with correction of hypotension in patients with multiple trauma for example, and eradication of any source of sepsis (e.g. intra-abdominal abscess or ischaemic bowel post-surgery).

Respiratory support

Characteristically the hypoxaemia of ARDS is refractory to **oxygen therapy** because of shunting of blood through areas of lung which are not being ventilated as a result of the alveoli being filled with a proteinaceous exudate and undergoing atelectasis. **Continuous positive airway pressure (CPAP)** can be applied via a tight-fitting nasal mask to prevent alveolar atelectasis and thereby reduce ventilation/perfusion mismatch and the work of breathing. However, **endotracheal intubation and mechanical ventilation** rapidly become nec-

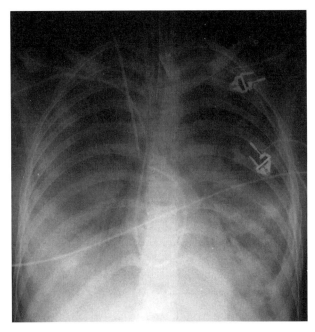

Fig. 18.2 This 21-year-old diabetic patient was admitted to the intensive therapy unit (ITU) having vomited and inhaled gastric contents while unconscious with severe ketoacidosis. Despite antibiotics and treatment of ketoacidosis she developed acute respiratory distress syndrome (ARDS) with progressive respiratory distress and severe hypoxaemia refractory to oxygen therapy. The chest X-ray shows diffuse bilateral shadowing with air bronchograms (black tubes of air against the white background of consolidated lung). An endotracheal tube is in place and the patient is being mechanically ventilated, with a positive end expiratory pressure (PEEP) of 7.5 cmH$_2$O. Electrocardiogram monitor leads are visible and a central venous line has been inserted via the right internal jugular vein. A Swan–Ganz catheter has been passed from the right subclavian vein and can be seen, looped around through the right side of the heart into the pulmonary artery. Pulmonary capillary wedge pressure was low at 8 mmHg indicating that the lung shadowing was not due to cardiogenic pulmonary oedema, but was due to increased capillary permeability of ARDS. Despite requiring prolonged ventilation and support on ITU the patient made a full recovery.

essary and the patient may need to be transferred to a **specialist intensive therapy unit (ITU)** with expertise and facilities for treating ARDS. Intermittent positive pressure ventilation mechanically inflates the lungs delivering oxygen-enriched air at a set tidal volume and rate. Adjustments in the volume, inflation pressure, rate and percentage oxygen are made to achieve adequate ventilation. A **positive end expiratory pressure (PEEP)** of 5–15 cmH$_2$O is usually applied at the end of the expiratory cycle to prevent collapse of the alveoli. High airway pressures may be generated in ventilating the non-compliant, stiff lungs in ARDS and this can reduce cardiac output and carries the risk of barotrauma (e.g. pneumothorax). High pressures combined with high oxygen concentrations may themselves result in microvascular damage which perpetuates the problem of permeability pulmonary oedema ('ventilator lung/oxygen toxicity'). A variety of ventilatory techniques have been developed to overcome these problems. **Inverse ratio ventilation** prolongs the inspiratory phase of ventilation such that it is longer than the expiratory phase allowing the tidal volume to be delivered over a longer time at a lower pressure. This may, however, cause progressive air trapping. **High-frequency jet ventilation** is a technique whereby small volumes are delivered as an injected jet of gas at high frequencies (e.g. 100–300 per minute). Ventilation of the patient in the **prone posture** may be beneficial as it reduces gravity-dependent fluid deposition and atelectasis. **Extra corporeal membrane oxygenation** (ECMO) involves the diversion of the patient's circulation through an artificial external membrane to provide oxygen and remove carbon dioxide. None of these ventilatory strategies has yet achieved a major improvement in the overall prognosis of ARDS but each may be useful in individual circumstances.

Optimizing haemodynamic function

Reducing the pulmonary artery pressure may help to reduce the degree of pulmonary capillary leak. This is achieved by avoiding excessive fluid administration, by judicious use of **diuretics** and by use of drugs which act as **vasodilators** of the pulmonary arteries. Treatment is often guided by use of a balloon-tipped pulmonary artery catheter (Swan–Ganz) which measures pulmonary artery pressures, pulmonary capillary wedge pressure (reflecting left atrial pressure) and cardiac output (using a thermal dilution technique). Haemodynamic management essentially consists of achieving an **optimal balance** between a **low pulmonary artery pressure** to reduce fluid leak to the alveoli, an **adequate systemic blood pressure** to maintain perfusion of tissues and organs (e.g. kidneys) with a satisfactory **cardiac output** and optimal **oxygen delivery** to tissues (oxygen delivery is a function of the haemoglobin level, oxygen saturation of blood and cardiac output). Most drugs used to vasodilate the pulmonary arteries, such as nitrates or calcium antagonists, also cause systemic vasodilatation with hypotension and impaired organ perfu-

sion. Inotropes and vasopressor agents, such as **dobutamine** or **noradrenaline** may be needed to maintain systemic blood pressure and cardiac output particularly in patients with the sepsis syndrome (caused by septicaemia or peritonitis, for example) in which sepsis is associated with systemic vasodilatation. Recently, inhaled **nitric oxide** (NO) has been used as a selective pulmonary artery vasodilator. Since it is given by inhalation it is selectively distributed to ventilated regions of the lung where it produces vasodilatation. This vasodilatation to ventilated alveoli may significantly improve ventilation/perfusion matching with improved gas exchange. Nitric oxide is rapidly inactivated by haemoglobin preventing a systemic action. It is necessary to monitor the level of inspired gas, nitrogen dioxide (NO_2) and methaemoglobin to avoid toxicity.

General management

Correction of anaemia by **blood transfusions** improves oxygen carriage in the blood and oxygen delivery to the tissues. **Nutritional support** (e.g. by enteral feeding via a jejunostomy) is crucial in maintaining the patient's overall fitness in the face of critical illness, and correction of hypoalbuminaemia improves the osmotic pressure of the plasma reducing fluid leak from the circulation. The ventilated patient with ARDS is particularly vulnerable to **nosocomial pneumonia** and bronchoalveolar lavage may be helpful in identifying pathogens. **Multi-organ failure** often complicates ARDS requiring further specific interventions (e.g. dialysis for renal failure).

Anti-inflammatory therapies

A key target for potential treatment is the cascade of inflammatory events arising from the tissue damage resulting from the initiating illness. Unfortunately these events are poorly understood and no anti-inflammatory drug has yet achieved an established role in treating ARDS. Corticosteroids have not been beneficial. Ibuprofen has been used in an attempt to reduce neutrophil activation and pentoxifylline has been used because of its action in reducing the production of interleukin-1. Haemofiltration is a procedure primarily used to control fluid balance but it may have an additional beneficial effect in patients with sepsis by removal of endotoxins.

Prognosis

Despite intensive research into the inflammatory mechanism giving rise to ARDS and major advances in ventilatory techniques and haemodynamic control the mortality of patients with ARDS remains very high at >50%. Patients who survive may be left with lung fibrosis and impaired gas diffusion but some patients make a remarkably full recovery despite having been critically ill with gross lung injury requiring prolonged treatment in ITU.

Further reading

Ashbaugh DG, Bigelow DB, Petty TL, Levine BE. Acute respiratory distress in adults. *Lancet* 1967; **ii**: 319–23.

Bernard GR, Artigas A, Brigham KL *et al.* Report of the American–European Consensus Conference on ARDS. *Intensive Care Med* 1994; **20**: 225–32.

Burchardi H. New strategies in mechanical ventilation for acute lung injury. *Eur Respir J* 1996; **9**: 1063–72.

Oh TE. Defining adult respiratory distress syndrome. *Br J Hosp Med* 1992; **47**: 350–3.

Tighe D, Moss R, Bennett D. The history of trauma and its relationship to the adult respiratory distress syndrome. *Br J Intensive Care* 1996; **6**: 272–4.

CHAPTER 19

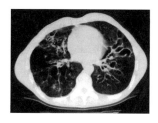

Sleep-Related Breathing Disorders

Introduction

People spend almost one-third of their lives asleep but it is only relatively recently that we have become aware of the important effects of sleep on respiratory physiology, and of specific breathing disorders occurring during sleep, such as the obstructive sleep apnoea syndrome.

Sleep physiology

Although familiar to everyone as a state in which the eyes are closed, postural muscles relaxed and consciousness suspended, sleep is an enigmatic condition which has essential refreshing and restorative effects on the mind and body. Electroencephalogram (EEG) studies show that sleep may be divided into five stages and two major categories. Stages 1–4 are characterized by loss of alpha wave activity and progressive slowing in the frequency with increase in the amplitude of the EEG wave form, and during these stages rapid eye movements are absent: **non-REM sleep**. Stage 5 is characterized by rapid eye movement: **REM sleep**. Typically a person drifts from an awake relaxed state into sleep, progressing serially through EEG stages 1–4, becoming less responsive to stimuli and less rousable. After about 70 minutes of non-REM sleep the person usually enters a period of deep sleep associated with rapid eye movements. This usually lasts about 30 minutes and is often followed by a brief awakening and a return to stage 1 sleep. Cycles of REM and non-REM sleep continue throughout the night with the period spent in REM sleep becoming longer, such that it occupies about 25% of total sleep time. During REM sleep the person is difficult to rouse and has reduced muscle tone. This stage of sleep is associated with dreaming and a variety of autonomic changes including penile erection and changes in respiration, blood pressure, pulse rate and pupil diameter. Irregularity of respiration and heart rate are common in this stage of sleep and apnoeic episodes lasting 15–20 seconds are common in normal individuals. The exact sleep 'architecture' (depth, character and changes) varies with age and circumstances (e.g. unfamiliar environment, disruption of regular routine), so that it can be difficult to define precisely normal and abnormal patterns by arbitrary cut-off points. Although sleep has major beneficial effects on the mind and body the physiological changes during sleep may aggravate pre-existing respiratory disease, and specific breathing disorders may arise during sleep.

Oxygen desaturation during sleep in respiratory disease

During sleep the respiratory centre in the medulla receives less stimulation from higher cortical centres and becomes less responsive to chemical (e.g. hypercapnia) and mechanical (e.g. from chest wall and airway receptors) stimuli. Minute ventilation (tidal volume and respiratory rate), falls, Pco_2 rises, functional residual capacity decreases and there is diminished activity of the intercostal and accessory respiratory muscles. These changes are most marked during REM sleep. Although they are not associated with any adverse effects in normal individuals they may produce profound nocturnal hypoxaemia and hypercapnia in patients with underlying respiratory disease, who are dependent on accessory respiratory muscle activity and who are already hypoxic when awake and on the steep part of the oxy-haemoglobin dissociation curve. Sleep-related oxygen desaturation is most important in diseases associated with hypercapnic (type 2) respiratory failure such as **chronic obstructive pulmonary disease (COPD)**, **neuromuscular disease** (e.g. muscular dystrophy, motor neurone disease) and **thoracic cage disorders** (e.g. kyphoscoliosis). The nocturnal oxygen desaturation in these disorders results from the deleterious effect of sleep physiology on pre-existing respiratory insufficiency and is quite distinct from obstructive sleep apnoea syndrome (see below).

Treatment

Optimizing the management of the **underlying respiratory disease** is the first priority (e.g. bronchodilators in COPD). Avoidance of **aggravating factors**, such as use of alcohol or sedative medication is important. Supplemental **oxygen** may alleviate oxygen desaturation but may provoke further hypoventilation and carbon dioxide retention since in many of these patients respiratory drive is partly dependent on the stimulant effect of hypoxaemia. **Protriptyline**, a non-sedative tricyclic antidepressant, may have a beneficial effect by reducing the time spent in REM sleep, but anti-cholinergic side-effects (e.g. dry mouth, urinary retention) are common.

There are very few drugs which have **respiratory stimulant** effects but an intravenous infusion of doxapram may be useful for a short period during a crisis. **Ventilatory support** can be delivered in the short term by endotracheal ventilation in an intensive therapy unit (ITU) to tide the patient over a crisis. However, long-term ventilatory support is often required and this is nowadays usually given as domiciliary nocturnal non-invasive **nasal intermittent positive pressure ventilation** (NIPPV). A tight-fitting mask is strapped in place over the nose and connected to a specifically designed ventilating machine. The spontaneous respiratory efforts of the patient trigger the ventilator to deliver additional tidal volume under positive pressure. Despite the cumbersome nature of this form of ventilatory support it is very well tolerated by patients who usually can manage to sleep whilst receiving nasal ventilation after a few nights of acclimatization. Control of nocturnal desaturation by NIPPV not only improves the quality of their sleep and nocturnal symptoms but also improves daytime symptoms and gas exchange. It seems that improvement of arterial blood gas levels during ventilation, resting fatigued respiratory muscles, recruiting atelectatic alveoli, relief of sleep deprivation and control of nocturnal hypoventilation by NIPPV all result in some recalibration of ventilatory responses with sustained improvement which ameliorates daytime gases also. NIPPV represents an important advance in the treatment of patients with ventilatory failure due to kyphoscoliosis, for example (Fig. 19.1).

Obstructive sleep apnoea syndrome (Fig. 19.2)

Obstructive sleep apnoea syndrome (OSAS) is a condition in which recurrent episodes of **upper airway occlusion** occur **during sleep** causing diminution (hypopnoea) or cessation of airflow **(apnoea)** in the pharynx provoking arousals and **sleep fragmentation**, resulting in daytime **sleepiness**.

Pathogenesis

The oropharyngeal dilator muscles play an important role in maintaining patency of the

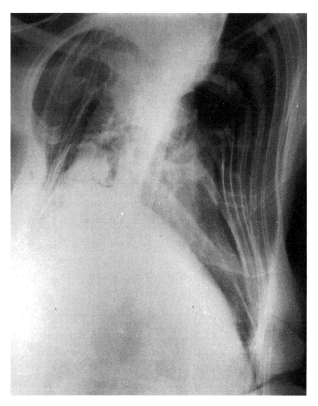

Fig. 19.1 This 39-year-old woman with severe kyphoscoliosis developed sleep disturbance, tiredness, headaches and oedema. She was erroneously treated with sedatives for insomnia. Spirometry showed a severe restrictive defect with forced expiratory volume in 1 second (FEV$_1$) of 0.4 and forced vital capacity (FVC) of 0.5 litre. Po$_2$ was 5.6 kPa (42 mmHg) and Pco$_2$ 10.2 kPa (76 mmHg). Her sleep was fragmented with multiple arousals and profound oxygen desaturation. She was unable to tolerate oxygen because of deteriorating hypercapnia. Nocturnal ventilatory support was commenced using non-invasive positive pressure ventilation (NIPPV) delivered via a tight nasal mask. She has now been using NIPPV for about 8 hours at night at home for 2 years. She works as a secretary and can do housework but is dyspnoeic on walking 150 metres. NIPPV is an effective means of ventilatory support for patients with hypercapnic respiratory failure due to thoracic cage disorders or neuromuscular disease.

upper airway. During deep sleep there is reduced muscle tone so that the pharyngeal airway is most vulnerable to collapse during REM sleep. Use of sedatives or alcohol may cause a further loss of muscle tone. Narrowing of the upper airway predisposes to occlusion and this is usually due to fat deposition in the neck from obesity, but other factors such as bone morphology (e.g. micrognathia), soft tissue deposition (e.g. hypothyroidism, acromegaly), or enlargement of tonsils or ade-noids in children may be important. Contraction of the diaphragm and intercostal muscles during inspiration creates a negative pressure in the airways drawing air into the lungs. The negative pressure in the airway, however, also acts as a force sucking in or collapsing the upper airway. An increase in upper airway resistance such as occurs in nasal obstruction (e.g. deviated nasal septum, polyps) or in enlargement of tonsils and adenoids, requires a greater inspiratory effort to overcome it, and

OBSTRUCTIVE SLEEP APNOEA

PATHOGENESIS

- (1) **Reduced calibre of pharyngeal airway**
  Obesity
  Micrognathia
  Acromegaly
  Hypothyroidism
  Large tonsils
  Large adenoids

- (2) **Reduced pharyngeal dilator muscle tone**
  REM sleep
  Sedatives
  Alcohol

- (3) **Inspiratory effort in increased upper airway resistance**
  Nasal polyps
  Deviated nasal septum
  Large tonsils
  Large adenoids

OROPHARYNGEAL
AIRWAY

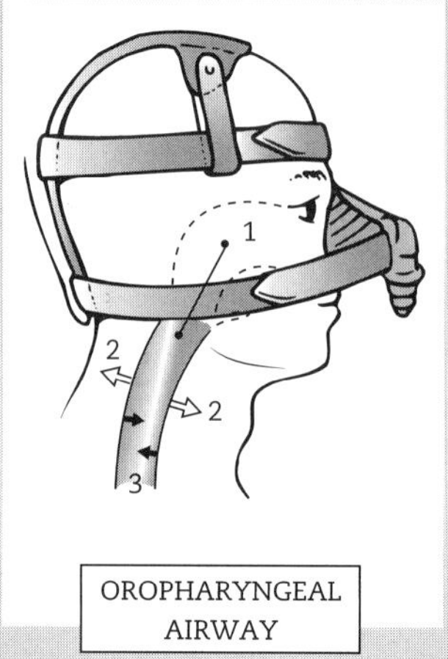

TREATMENT

- **General measures**
  Weight loss
  Avoid alcohol
  Avoid sedatives

- **Drugs**
  Protriptyline
  Acetazolamide
  Progesterone

- **Nasal CPAP**

- **Surgery**
  Tonsillectomy
  Nasal septum surgery
  Uvulopalatopharyngoplasty
  Tracheostomy
  Mandibular advancement

Fig. 19.2 Apnoea results from occlusion of pharyngeal airway in patients with narrowed airways when there is loss of pharyngeal dilator muscle tone in sleep. Increased inspiratory effort, when there is increased upper airway resistance, 'sucks in' the pharyngeal airway. Nasal continuous positive airway pressure (CPAP) acts as a splint preventing collapse of the airway and is the main treatment used for sleep apnoea.

thus increases the forces sucking in the pharyngeal airway. Although upper airway reflexes and neuromuscular control of respiration may also be important the main factors involved in upper airway patency are the **calibre of the pharyngeal airway**, the action of **oropharyngeal dilator muscles** and the **inspiratory effort** needed to overcome **upper airway resistance**.

OSAS is characterized by recurrent episodes of pharyngeal airway obstruction during sleep with apnoea, arousal and sleep fragmentation. As the patient with a compromised pharyngeal airway (e.g. narrowed by obesity) enters deep sleep the reduction in oropharyngeal dilator muscle tone results in collapse of the airway causing apnoea (cessa-

tion of airflow) or hypopnoea (reduction of airflow) with a fall in oxygen saturation. Inspiratory effort increases as the diaphragm and intercostal muscles try to overcome the closed upper airway. The apnoea is terminated by a brief arousal from sleep and this is associated with a burst of sympathetic nerve activity, release of catecholamines and fluctuations in pulse rate and blood pressure. Resumption of pharyngeal airflow is accompanied by loud snoring which is an inspiratory noise arising from vibration of the soft tissues of the oropharynx. Arousals are often associated with generalized body movement. Hundreds of episodes of apnoea and arousal throughout the night disrupt sleep, resulting in daytime sleepiness.

Clinical features

Patients with OSAS may have no detectable respiratory abnormality when awake but *daytime symptoms* include excessive **sleepiness**, **poor concentration**, **irritability**, **morning headaches** and **loss of libido**. It is important to recognize the relationship of such symptoms to sleep. The sleepiness is usually severe and results in **road traffic accidents** from falling asleep when driving, for example. The patient may be unaware of *night-time symptoms* but the bed partner may report loud **snoring**, witnessed **apnoeas** and **restless sleep**. It is important to enquire about use of sedatives or alcohol which may aggravate OSAS. *Examination* focuses on risk factors for OSAS such as **obesity**, **increased neck circumference**, anatomical abnormalities reducing **pharyngeal calibre** (e.g. micrognathia, enlarged tonsils), and **nasal obstruction** (e.g. polyps, deviated septum).

OSAS is associated with an increased incidence of **cardiovascular diseases** such as hypertension, myocardial infarction and cerebrovascular accidents. It has been suggested that this relates to the cardiovascular response to catecholamine release during apnoeas and arousals, but the evidence is inconclusive and it is difficult to separate the influence of OSAS from concomitant cardiovascular risk factors in these patients who are usually obese. It is important to reduce cardiovascular risk factors in these patients by checking smoking history, blood pressure, and cholesterol and glucose levels, and intervening as appropriate. In addition to catecholamine release, OSAS is associated with other **hormonal changes** including reduced testosterone and growth hormone levels. Although hypoxaemia, hypercapnia, and elevation of pulmonary artery pressure occur during apnoeas, cor pulmonale is unusual unless there is concomitant lung disease (e.g. COPD). The long-term prognosis of OSAS is not fully understood but some studies have shown a significantly higher mortality in patients who refused treatment than in those whose sleep apnoea was controlled by continuous positive airway pressure (CPAP).

Polysomnography

Although OSAS may sometimes be diagnosed on the basis of clinical features and overnight oximetry, definitive assessment requires polysomnography. This involves the recording of signals relating to oxygenation, airflow, chest wall movement and stage of sleep. An **electroencephalogram (EEG)** records the stage of sleep. An **electro-oculogram (EOG)** detects rapid eye movement. A thermistor detects **airflow** at the nose and mouth, and **ribcage** and **abdominal movements** are measured using magnetometers or impedance plethysmography. **Oximetry** detects oxygen desaturation and an **electrocardiogram (ECG)** records heart rate. These tracings are often combined with a video recording of the patient during sleep which permits observation of the patient's position and movement in relation to apnoeas and arousals.

The number of apnoeas increases with age and there is a continuum from normality to full-blown OSAS, so that it is difficult to define precise diagnostic criteria. However, OSAS is usually diagnosed when there are more than 10 apnoeas or hypopnoeas per hour: **apnoea/hypopnoea index >10**. These are usually associated with **oxygen desaturation of >4%**. For OSAS to be regarded as clinically significant, requiring treatment, the patient should have typical symptoms (e.g. daytime sleepiness) combined with an apnoea hypopnoea index > 10. Using these criteria about 4% of middle-aged men have OSAS.

Treatment

• *General measures*: **weight loss** is the most important treatment for most patients, although it is difficult to achieve. Even a small loss in weight can result in a significant improvement with a 10% reduction in weight typically resulting in a 50% improvement in the apnoea/hypopnoea index. Dietary advice, increased exercise and behavioural modification are crucial in achieving and maintaining weight reduction. Aggravating factors should be removed by **avoidance of alcohol and sedatives** before sleep. Snoring and OSAS are more common when the patient sleeps lying on his or her back so that sometimes measures such as sewing a tennis ball onto the back of the pyjamas **discourage sleeping on the back**. Tonsillectomy, excision of nasal polyps or correction of a deviated nasal septum may be appropriate in some cases. Attention should also be directed towards eliminating any concomitant risk factors for cardiovascular disease. Any underlying lung disease (e.g. COPD) should be treated appropriately.

• *Pharmacological treatments*: a number of drugs have a potential role in treating OSAS but none is particularly effective. **Protriptylline** is a non-sedative anti-depressant which reduces the time spent in REM sleep. **Progesterone** has some effect in stimulating respiratory drive. **Acetazolamide** enhances ventilatory drive by producing a metabolic acidosis through inhibition of renal tubular secretion of hydrogen ion.

• *Nasal CPAP* (e.g. 5–15 cmH$_2$O) applied via a tight-fitting **nasal mask** has become the standard treatment for OSAS. It is very effective and acts by splinting the pharyngeal airway open, counteracting the tendency to airway collapse. It is, however, a cumbersome treatment and some patients show poor compliance with this treatment in the long term.

• *Surgery*:   **uvulopalatopharyngoplasty** (UPPP) involves the surgical excision of redundant tissue of the soft palate, uvula and pharyngeal walls in order to increase the calibre of the pharyngeal airway. It is effective in stopping snoring but its effect on sleep apnoea is unpredictable and where beneficial the effect is often short-lived. Side-effects include post-operative pain, changes in the quality of the voice and sometimes nasal regurgitation during swallowing. **Tracheostomy** is effective but is a treatment of last resort. Surgical correction of bone abnormalities, such as **mandibular advancement** for micrognathia, can be effective in

appropriate cases. The lower jaw may be held in an open, slightly advanced position by the use of specifically designed **dental devices** but this may have an adverse effect on the temporomandibular joint in the long term.

Central sleep apnoea

Central sleep apnoea is a rare, poorly understood condition in which sleep-related apnoeas occur due to an apparent **lack of ventilatory drive** from the respiratory centres in the medulla. Polysomnography shows that cessation of airflow at the nose and mouth is associated with a lack of respiratory muscle activity. Sometimes obstructive sleep apnoea seems to provoke reflex inhibition of inspiratory drive so that central apnoeas follow classic obstructive apnoeas. Patients with this reflex central apnoea respond to nasal CPAP. Primary central sleep apnoea is rare but may result from instability of respiratory drive due to damage to the respiratory centres by brainstem infarcts or syringobulbia, for example. Most of these patients also have hypercapnic respiratory failure when awake, and nasal intermittent positive pressure ventilation is the main form of treatment used.

Further reading

De Backer WA. Central sleep apnoea, pathogenesis and treatment. *Eur Respir J* 1995; **8**: 1372–83.

Griffiths CJ, Cooper BG, Gibson GJ. A video system for investigating breathing disorders during sleep. *Thorax* 1991; **46**: 136–40.

Hudgel DW. Treatment of obstructive sleep apnoea. *Chest* 1996; **109**: 1346–58.

McNicholas WT. Impact of sleep in respiratory failure. *Eur Respir J* 1997; **10**: 920–33.

Strohl KP, Redline S. Recognition of obstructive sleep apnoea. *Am J Respir Crit Care Med* 1996; **154**: 279–89.

CHAPTER 20

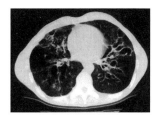

Lung Transplantation

Introduction

Replacement of diseased lungs by healthy donor lungs is the ultimate treatment option for patients with advanced lung disease not amenable to other forms of treatment. However, lung transplantation is associated with a high mortality and an uncertain long-term prognosis, and the lack of donor organs severely limits the application of the procedure. The first heart transplantation was performed in 1967 in Groote Schuur hospital, South Africa, when a man in end-stage cardiac failure received the heart of a young woman killed in a road traffic accident. Initial attempts at lung transplantation were fraught with difficulties and it was not until 1981 that the first successful heart–lung transplantation was performed in Stanford, USA, for a patient with primary pulmonary hypertension.

Types of operation

Surgical techniques have been developed to transplant a single lung, both lungs or the heart and lungs.

Heart–lung transplant

The recipient's diseased lungs and heart are removed through a median sternotomy and the donor lungs and heart are implanted as a block. If the recipient's heart is normal it may be donated to another patient (domino procedure).

Single-lung transplant

A diseased lung is removed through a thoracotomy incision whilst leaving the heart and contralateral lung intact. The donor lung is then implanted using a bronchial anastomosis. The residual native lung must be free of infection or it will be a source of sepsis in the post-operative period when the patient is immuno-suppressed, so that this procedure is not suitable for patients with cystic fibrosis, for example. The donor's heart and other lung are available to transplant to other patients.

Bilateral lung transplant

• *Double lung transplant*: the diseased lungs are removed through a median sternotomy whilst leaving the heart intact. The donor lungs are implanted as a block using a tracheal anastomosis.

• *Bilateral sequential single lung transplant*: a transverse bilateral thoracotomy is performed dividing the sternum horizontally. The diseased lungs are removed and two separated lungs are implanted with separate bronchial anastomoses.

Donor organs are most commonly procured from young adults involved in road traffic accidents and ventilated on intensive therapy units, who are then diagnosed as having suffered brain-stem death. There are strict guidelines governing the diagnosis of brain-stem death and the process of organ donation. Because of the vulnerability of the lungs to injury and infection only about 20% of suitable heart donors will also be potential lung donors. There must be no history of significant respiratory disease and no major chest trauma. Chest X-ray must be clear and gas exchange adequate ($P_{O_2} > 12$ kPa (90 mmHg) on $<35\%$ inspired oxygen). Techniques have been developed to preserve the donor lungs for up to 8 hours allowing emergency transport (e.g. by plane) of donor organs to the recipient. The donor and recipient are matched for ABO blood group, cytomegalovirus status and chest size.

Indications for transplantation

Although in theory many types of end-stage lung disease would be amenable to transplantation, in practice the lack of donor organs severely restricts the procedure. Lung transplantation has proved a successful treatment for patients with cystic fibrosis, primary pulmonary hypertension, emphysema due to α_1-anti-trypsin deficiency, cryptogenic fibrosing alveolitis, and a variety of rare diseases such as eosinophilic granuloma. The patient should be **ill enough to need a lung transplant** but **not so ill as to be unable to withstand** the surgery. Furthermore, the patient must be aware of the risks and benefits of transplantation and must actively **want to undergo** the operation. In patients with cystic fibrosis, for example, a forced expiratory volume in 1 second (FEV_1) $< 30\%$ predicted, a $P_{O_2} < 7.5$ kPa (55 mmHg) and a $P_{CO_2} > 6.5$ kPa (50 mmHg) are associated with a 50% mortality within 2 years, and it is at this stage that lung transplantation should be considered (Fig. 20.1). The patient needs time to understand the severity

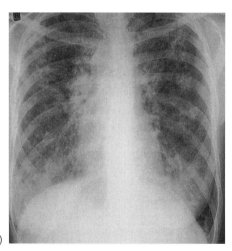 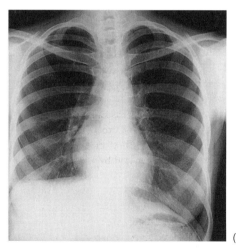

(a)   (b)

Fig. 20.1 This 29-year-old woman developed respiratory failure (P_{O_2} 6 kPa (45 mmHg), P_{CO_2} 8 kPa (60 mmHg)) due to advanced cystic fibrosis lung disease (forced expiratory volume in 1 second (FEV_1) 0.5 litre). Her chest X-ray (a) shows hyperinflated lungs with diffuse bronchiectasis and peribronchial fibrosis. She was accepted onto a lung transplantation waiting list and supported by oxygen therapy, antibiotics, physiotherapy and nutritional supplements whilst awaiting donor lungs. Her hypercapnic respiratory failure deteriorated and she was 'bridged' to transplantation by domiciliary intermittent positive pressure ventilation delivered via a tight-fitting nasal mask. Bilateral sequential single-lung transplantations were performed (b) 14 months after being accepted onto the waiting list. Two years after transplantation she was very well but had evidence of early obliterative bronchiolitis.

of the disease, the predicted prognosis and what is involved in lung transplantation. Addressing these issues is traumatic for the patient and his or her family. Some patients with advanced lung disease want to try all available treatment options whereas other patients fear high-intensity unpleasant interventions and would prefer to take a palliative approach to the terminal stages of their disease. **Contra-indications** to lung transplantation include **hepatic** or **renal disease**, **uncontrolled infection**, the presence of an **aspergilloma** and **poor nutritional** status. The success of lung transplantation programmes is based upon careful selection of the small number of patients who can benefit from the procedure and who can be supported long enough to have a realistic chance of getting a donor organ.

Post-transplantation complications and treatment

In the first few days post-transplantation **reimplantation injury** may occur with infiltrates developing in the donor lung as a result of increased capillary permeability due to surgical trauma, ischaemia, denervation and lymphatic interruption. Early post-operative **surgical complications** include haemorrhage and dehiscence of the anastomosis. Prophylactic antibiotics are given to counter **'donor-acquired' infection** since the donor lungs are often contaminated by bacteria. Lavage of the donor organ is performed before implantation to identify infection. Intense **immunosuppression**, using a combination of cyclosporin, azathioprine and corticosteroids, is needed to prevent rejection of the donor lungs. Anti-thymocyte globulin may be given for the first few days to suppress further T-cell function. Patients remain on cyclosporin and azathioprine indefinitely and are at ongoing risk from two particular hazards: **rejection** and **infection**. Both may present with similar clinical features of malaise, pyrexia, infiltrates on chest X-ray, impaired oxygenation and reduced lung function. Bronchoscopy, with bron-

choalveolar lavage and transbronchial biopsy are the key investigations in identifying rejection of the donor lung and infection. Episodes of **acute rejection** are treated by intensification of immunosuppression, e.g. intravenous methylprednisolone, sometimes with monoclonal T-cell antibody (OKT_3). The treatment of infection is crucially dependent upon identification of the causative organism since the patient is at risk from both bacterial and **opportunistic infections**, e.g. *Pneumocystis carinii*, cytomegalovirus or fungi (see Chapter 8). *Pneumocystis carinii* prophylaxis (e.g. septrin) is given routinely. **Lymphoproliferative disorders** such as Epstein–Barr-virus-related B-cell lymphoma may develop as a result of immunosuppression. Treatment consists of acyclovir with a reduction in immunosuppression. **Obliterative bronchiolitis** is the most important complication threatening the long-term survival of patients after lung transplantation. It results from chronic rejection of the donor lungs and is characterized by progressive airways obstruction due to obliteration of the bronchioles by organizing fibrosis. **Recurrence of the primary disease** in the donor lungs has been documented in recipients with sarcoidosis but the outcome has not been affected by this in most cases.

Prognosis

The mortality rate after lung transplantation is about 15% at 1 month, 30% at 1 year and 40% at 3 years. The quality of life of the patients is dramatically improved by a successful lung transplantation but the long-term prognosis is limited particularly by the occurrence of obliterative bronchiolitis. This and the shortage of donor organs remain the two main problems to be overcome.

Further reading

Corris PA. Post heart/lung transplantation management. *J R Soc Med* 1995; **88** (Suppl. 25): 37–40.
Heritier F, Madden B, Hodson ME, Yacoub M. Lung

allograft transplantation: indications, preoperative assessment and postoperative management. *Eur Respir J* 1992; **5**: 1262–78.

Kotloff RM, Zuckerman JB. Lung transplantation for cystic fibrosis: special considerations. *Chest* 1996; **109**: 787–98.

Levine SM, Gibbons WJ, Bryan CL *et al.* Single lung transplantation for primary pulmonary hypertension. *Chest* 1990; **98**: 1107–15.

Trulock EP. Lung transplantation. *Am J Respir Crit Care Med* 1997; **155**: 789–818.

Index

dust (*cont.*)
  environmental   139
  inhaled   148
  iron   153
  see also occupational lung disease
dyspnoea   8
  paroxysmal nocturnal   8

elastic recoil   4, *114*
electrocardiogram, pulmonary embolism   159
emphysema   113, *114*, 115
  α_1 antitrypsin deficiency
  airflow obstruction   112
  centriacinar   113
  coalworker's   153
  panacinar   115
empyema   48, 174
  drainage   175
  tuberculosis   175
endotracheal intubation   179
environment
  asthma   92, 93
    indoor environment   93
    outdoor environment   93
  lung cancer   **128**
  occupational lung disease   14
  pneumonia   49
eosinophilia   75, 95, 165
epiglottitis   *42*, 44
Epstein–Barr virus   42, 191
  AIDS   70
erythema nodosum   *144*
erythromycin   52–4
ethambutol   61, 64
examination of respiratory system   11–15, *16*, *17*
exercise in asthma   99–100, 104
exercise training in COPD   122
  non-maximal   23
extracorporeal membrane oxygenation (ECMO)   181
extrinsic allergic alveolitis   143
exudates   *172*, 174

family history   10
farmer's lung   143
fat embolism   164
fibrinolysis   159
fibrosing alveolitis
  cryptogenic   139–41, *141*
    clinical course   140–1
    histological features   139–40
    mortality   141
    treatment   141
  rheumatoid disease   141
  systemic lupus erythematosus   142

systemic sclerosis   142
fibrosis   34, 37
  asbestosis   154
  diffuse interstitial   *140*
  inhaled dust   148
  intra-alveolar buds of organizing   142
  lung cancer incidence   127
  pneumoconiosis   151, *152*
flax   151
flow meter   *20*
flow–volume loop   20–1, 24, *26*
flucloxacillin   53, 87
fluoroscopy   24
fluticasone   105
forced expiratory spirogram   19, *22*
forced expiratory volume in 1 second (FEV$_1$)   20, *22*
forced vital capacity (FVC)   19, *22*
foreign body   73, 97
fossil fuels   94
functional residual capacity   18, *19*
fungal infections
  AIDS   70
  immunocompromised patients   72
  see also aspergillosis
fungal spores   93
Fusobacterium necrophorum   80

gas exchange   4–6
gastro-oesophageal reflux   9
Gastrografin swallow   50
genotyping, cystic fibrosis   86
glandular fever *see* infectious mononucleosis
goblet cells   3
Gohn focus   56
Goodpasture's syndrome   165–6
granuloma
  sarcoidosis   143
  tuberculosis   60
  Wegener's   165

β-haemolytic streptococci   41, 42
Haemophilus influenzae   41, *42*, 116
  bronchiectasis   78
  bronchitis exacerbation   46
  COPD   120
  cystic fibrosis   83
  non-typeable unencapsulated   52–3
  pneumonia   48, 52–3
  type b   44, 52
haemoptysis   9, **10**
  bronchiectasis   76
  cystic fibrosis   84
  lung abscess   79
  lung carcinoma   *130*
haemothorax   171